300

Full Body Kettlebell Workouts Book for Men and Women

300

Full Body Kettlebell Workouts Book for Men and Women

Guide to 150 Kettlebell Exercises & 150 Kettlebell & Bodyweight Exercises with Step-by-Step Guides & Images for Muscle Building & Fat Loss

Be.Bull Publishing Group

Authors:

Be.Bull Publishing Group

Mauricio Vasquez

First Printing: July 2024

ISBN-978-1-998402-59-5 (Paperback)
ISBN-978-1-998402-60-1 (Hardcover)

TIPS

- Adjust the number of repetitions and the time cap for the workouts according to your capabilities, skills and physical condition
- Listen to your body and don't push yourself too hard
- If you don't have enough space where to run, you can do jumping jacks. 100-meter run is approximately equivalent to 50 jumping jacks
- Walk into the gym with a workout already selected for you
- Get motivated with a fun workout playlist
- Put your phone on airplane mode
- Start your workout with some stretches
- Log the details of each workout so you can track your progress. You can track time and number of repetitions
- Enjoy your workouts

Dear valued customer,

Your opinion matters!

By leaving a review using the QR code provided, you can help fellow readers discover and enjoy this book. Your feedback will guide others in making informed decisions and enhance their reading experience.

Thank you for contributing to our reading community!

Mauricio

<u>Disclaimer</u>

FREE DOWNLOAD

BONUS No 1 - 1000 Full-Body Workouts

To access extra 1,000 workouts to stay motivated and avoid workout boredom with endless variety, scan this QR code:

BONUS No 2- Logging Sheets of Your Workout Book

To access your free e-copy of this workout book, scan this QR code:

If you want to add more variety to your workouts, scan this QR code to check these workout books!

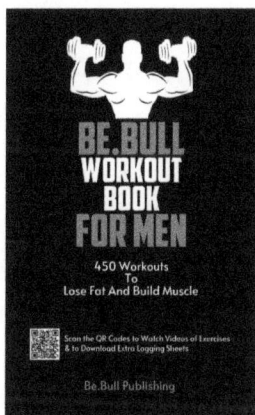

BE.BULL
WORKOUT
BOOK
FOR MEN

450 Workouts
To
Lose Fat And Build Muscle

Scan the QR Codes to Watch Videos of Exercises
& to Download Extra Logging Sheets

Be.Bull Publishing

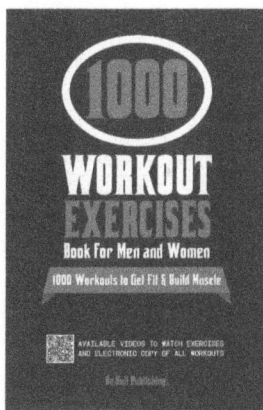

1000
WORKOUT
EXERCISES
Book For Men and Women
1000 Workouts to Get Fit & Build Muscle

AVAILABLE VIDEOS TO WATCH EXERCISES
AND ELECTRONIC COPY OF ALL WORKOUTS

Be.Bull Publishing

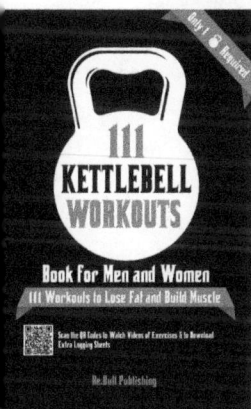

Only 1 Required

111
KETTLEBELL
WORKOUTS

Book For Men and Women
111 Workouts to Lose Fat and Build Muscle

Scan the QR Codes to Watch Videos of Exercises & to Download
Extra Logging Sheets

Be.Bull Publishing

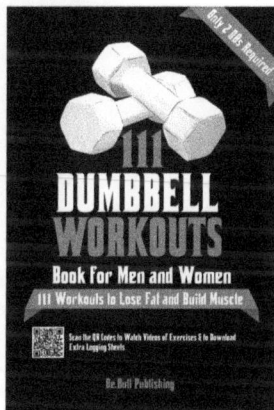

Only 2 lbs Required

111
DUMBBELL
WORKOUTS

Book For Men and Women
111 Workouts to Lose Fat and Build Muscle

Scan the QR Codes to Watch Videos of Exercises & to Download
Extra Logging Sheets

Be.Bull Publishing

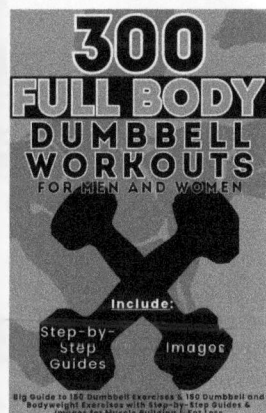

300
FULL BODY
DUMBBELL
WORKOUTS
FOR MEN AND WOMEN

Include:

Step-by-Step
Guides   Images

Big Guide to 150 Dumbbell Exercises & 150 Dumbbell and
Bodyweight Exercises with Step-by-Step Guides &
Images for Muscle Building & Fat Loss

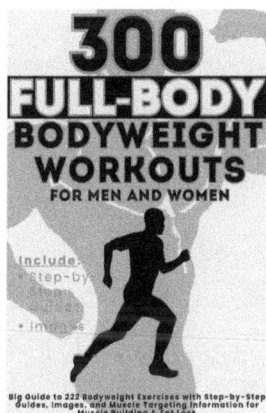

300
FULL-BODY
BODYWEIGHT
WORKOUTS
FOR MEN AND WOMEN

Include:
Step-by-
Step
Guides
Images

Big Guide to 222 Bodyweight Exercises with Step-by-Step
Guides, Images, and Muscle Targeting Information for
Muscle Building & Fat Loss

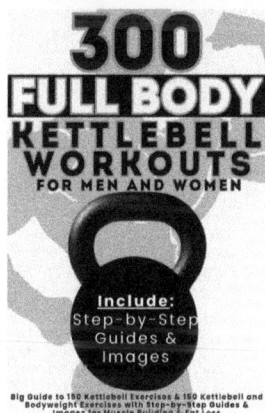

300
FULL BODY
KETTLEBELL
WORKOUTS
FOR MEN AND WOMEN

Include:
Step-by-Step
Guides &
Images

Big Guide to 150 Kettlebell Exercises & 150 Kettlebell and
Bodyweight Exercises with Step-by-Step Guides &
Images for Muscle Building & Fat Loss

Workout No.	Workout (Kettlebell & Body-Weight Workouts)	Main Muscle Groups	Instructions
	Repeat 4 times with 1-minute rest between rounds:		
1	(1) 30 seconds Kettlebell Swing	Lower Body, Core, Shoulders	Swing kettlebell between legs, thrust hips forward, raise kettlebell to shoulder height. Repeat for 30 seconds.
	(2) 30 seconds Burpees	Full Body, Core, Legs	Jump, squat down, kick back into push-up, return up. Repeat for 30 seconds.
	(3) 30 seconds Goblet Squat	Legs, Core, Glutes	Squat holding kettlebell close to chest, keep back straight. Repeat for 30 seconds.
	(4) 30 seconds High Knees	Legs, Cardio, Core	Run in place lifting knees high, maintain fast pace. Repeat for 30 seconds.
	3 Rounds for time:		
2	(1) 15 Kettlebell Clean and Press	Shoulders, Arms, Core	Clean kettlebell to shoulder, press overhead. Alternate arms. Complete 15 reps each arm.
	(2) 20 Push-Ups	Chest, Triceps, Core	Lower body to ground, push up with arms. Repeat for 20 reps.
	(3) 20 Kettlebell Goblet Squat	Legs, Glutes, Core	Squat holding kettlebell close to chest. Repeat for 20 reps.
	(4) 400-meter run	Legs, Cardio, Core	Run 400 meters at a steady pace.
	Repeat 5 times::		
3	(1) 40 seconds Kettlebell Snatch	Shoulders, Back, Core	Lift kettlebell overhead in one motion, lock arm. Alternate arms. Repeat for 40 seconds.
	(2) 20 seconds Rest		Rest for 20 seconds.
	(3) 40 seconds Mountain Climbers	Cardio, Core, Legs	Run in place in plank position, drive knees to chest. Repeat for 40 seconds.
	(4) 20 seconds Rest		Rest for 20 seconds.
	As many rounds as possible in 12 mins of:		
4	(1) 10 Kettlebell Deadlifts	Lower Back, Hamstrings, Glutes	Lift kettlebell from ground, keep back straight. Repeat for 10 reps.
	(2) 15 Box Jumps	Legs, Cardio, Core	Jump onto and off a box repeatedly. Repeat for 15 reps.
	(3) 20 Kettlebell Thrusters	Shoulders, Legs, Core	Squat to overhead press in one fluid motion. Repeat for 20 reps.
	(4) 25 Sit-Ups	Abs, Core, Hip Flexors	Perform sit-ups lying on back, hands behind head. Repeat for 25 reps.
	Repeat 4 times with 1-minute rest between rounds:		
5	(1) 30 seconds Single Arm Kettlebell Swing	Shoulders, Back, Core	Swing kettlebell with one hand, switch hands mid-air. Repeat for 30 seconds.
	(2) 30 seconds Jumping Jacks	Cardio, Legs, Core	Jump to spread legs and clap hands overhead. Repeat for 30 seconds.
	(3) 30 seconds Kettlebell Front Raise	Shoulders, Arms, Core	Lift kettlebell to shoulder height, keep arms straight. Repeat for 30 seconds.
	(4) 30 seconds Push-Ups	Chest, Triceps, Core	Lower body to ground, push up with arms. Repeat for 30 seconds.

Workout No.	Workout (Kettlebell & Body-Weight Workouts)	Main Muscle Groups	Instructions
	4 Rounds for time:		
	(1) 20 Kettlebell Swings	Lower Body, Core, Shoulders	Swing kettlebell between legs, thrust hips forward. Repeat for 20 reps.
6	(2) 20 Lunges	Legs, Glutes, Core	Step forward, lower hips to drop knee to ground. Repeat for 20 reps.
	(3) 15 Kettlebell Bent Over Rows	Back, Shoulders, Arms	Hinge forward, row kettlebell to hip. Repeat for 15 reps each side.
	(4) 200-meter run	Legs, Cardio, Core	Run 200 meters at a steady pace.
	Repeat 5 times:		
	(1) 45 seconds Kettlebell Around the Body	Core, Shoulders, Arms	Pass kettlebell around body, maintain core control. Repeat for 45 seconds.
7	(2) 15 seconds Rest		Rest for 15 seconds.
	(3) 45 seconds Burpees	Full Body, Core, Legs	Jump, squat down, kick back into push-up, return up. Repeat for 45 seconds.
	(4) 15 seconds Rest		Rest for 15 seconds.
	3 Rounds for time:		
	(1) 10 Kettlebell Snatches	Shoulders, Back, Core	Lift kettlebell overhead in one motion, lock arm. Alternate arms. Complete 10 reps each arm.
8	(2) 20 Air Squats	Legs, Glutes, Core	Stand, bend knees to lower body. Repeat for 20 reps.
	(3) 15 Kettlebell Deadlifts	Lower Back, Hamstrings, Glutes	Lift kettlebell from ground, keep back straight. Repeat for 15 reps.
	(4) 300-meter run	Legs, Cardio, Core	Run 300 meters at a steady pace.
	Repeat 8 times:		
	(1) 20 seconds Kettlebell Jump Swing	Legs, Core, Shoulders	Explosive swing with a jump at top of motion. Repeat for 20 seconds.
9	(2) 10 seconds Rest		Rest for 10 seconds.
	(3) 20 seconds Push-Up with Extension	Chest, Triceps, Core	Perform push-up, extend one arm forward. Repeat for 20 seconds.
	(4) 10 seconds Rest		Rest for 10 seconds.
	4 Rounds for time:		
	(1) 15 Kettlebell Clean	Shoulders, Back, Core	Lift kettlebell to shoulder, flip grip at top. Repeat for 15 reps.
10	(2) 20 V-Ups	Abs, Core, Hip Flexors	Lie back, lift legs and torso simultaneously. Repeat for 20 reps.
	(3) 20 Kettlebell Goblet Squat	Legs, Glutes, Core	Squat holding kettlebell close to chest. Repeat for 20 reps.
	(4) 250-meter run	Legs, Cardio, Core	Run 250 meters at a steady pace.

Workout No.	Workout (Kettlebell & Body-Weight Workouts)	Main Muscle Groups	Instructions
	3 Rounds for time:		
11	(1) 10 Kettlebell Deadlifts	Lower Back, Hamstrings, Glutes	Lift kettlebell from ground, keep back straight. Repeat for 10 reps.
	(2) 15 Push-Ups	Chest, Triceps, Core	Lower body to ground, push up with arms. Repeat for 15 reps.
	(3) 20 Kettlebell Goblet Squats	Legs, Glutes, Core	Squat holding kettlebell close to chest. Repeat for 20 reps.
	(4) 200-meter run	Legs, Cardio, Core	Run 200 meters at a steady pace.
	Repeat 4 times with 1-minute rest between rounds:		
12	(1) 30 seconds Kettlebell Swing	Lower Body, Core, Shoulders	Swing kettlebell between legs, thrust hips forward, raise kettlebell to shoulder height. Repeat for 30 seconds.
	(2) 30 seconds Mountain Climbers	Cardio, Core, Legs	Run in place in plank position, drive knees to chest. Repeat for 30 seconds.
	(3) 30 seconds Kettlebell Thrusters	Shoulders, Legs, Core	Squat to overhead press in one fluid motion. Repeat for 30 seconds.
	(4) 30 seconds Jumping Jacks	Cardio, Legs, Core	Jump to spread legs and clap hands overhead. Repeat for 30 seconds.
	3 Rounds for time:		
13	(1) 15 Kettlebell Clean and Press	Shoulders, Arms, Core	Clean kettlebell to shoulder, press overhead. Alternate arms. Complete 15 reps each arm.
	(2) 20 Air Squats	Legs, Glutes, Core	Stand, bend knees to lower body. Repeat for 20 reps.
	(3) 15 Kettlebell Bent Over Rows	Back, Shoulders, Arms	Hinge forward, row kettlebell to hip. Repeat for 15 reps each side.
	(4) 400-meter run	Legs, Cardio, Core	Run 400 meters at a steady pace.
	3 Rounds for time:		
14	(1) 15 Kettlebell Clean and Press	Shoulders, Back, Core	Clean kettlebell to shoulder, press overhead. Alternate arms. Complete 15 reps each arm.
	(2) 20 Air Squats		Stand, bend knees to lower body. Repeat for 20 reps.
	(3) 15 Kettlebell Bent Over Rows	Full Body, Core, Legs	Hinge forward, row kettlebell to hip. Repeat for 15 reps each side.
	(4) 400-meter run		Run 400 meters at a steady pace.
	4 Rounds for time:		
15	(1) 20 Kettlebell Swings	Lower Body, Core, Shoulders	Swing kettlebell between legs, thrust hips forward. Repeat for 20 reps.
	(2) 20 Lunges	Legs, Glutes, Core	Step forward, lower hips to drop knee to ground. Repeat for 20 reps.
	(3) 15 Kettlebell Shoulder Press	Shoulders, Arms, Core	Press kettlebell overhead from shoulder level. Repeat for 15 reps each side.
	(4) 200-meter run	Legs, Cardio, Core	Run 200 meters at a steady pace.

Workout No.	Workout (Kettlebell & Body-Weight Workouts)	Main Muscle Groups	Instructions
	Repeat 5 times:		
16	(1) 45 seconds Kettlebell Around the Body	Core, Shoulders, Arms	Pass kettlebell around body, maintain core control. Repeat for 45 seconds.
	(2) 15 seconds Rest		Rest for 15 seconds.
	(3) 45 seconds Jumping Jacks	Cardio, Legs, Core	Jump to spread legs and clap hands overhead. Repeat for 45 seconds.
	(4) 15 seconds Rest		Rest for 15 seconds.
	3 Rounds for time:		
17	(1) 10 Kettlebell Snatches	Shoulders, Back, Core	Lift kettlebell overhead in one motion, lock arm. Alternate arms. Complete 10 reps each arm.
	(2) 20 Push-Ups	Chest, Triceps, Core	Lower body to ground, push up with arms. Repeat for 20 reps.
	(3) 15 Kettlebell Deadlifts	Lower Back, Hamstrings, Glutes	Lift kettlebell from ground, keep back straight. Repeat for 15 reps.
	(4) 300-meter run	Legs, Cardio, Core	Run 300 meters at a steady pace.
	Repeat 8 times:		
18	(1) 20 seconds Kettlebell Jump Swing	Legs, Core, Shoulders	Explosive swing with a jump at top of motion. Repeat for 20 seconds.
	(2) 10 seconds Rest		Rest for 10 seconds.
	(3) 20 seconds High Knees	Legs, Cardio, Core	Run in place lifting knees high. Repeat for 20 seconds.
	(4) 10 seconds Rest		Rest for 10 seconds.
	4 Rounds for time:		
19	(1) 15 Kettlebell Clean	Shoulders, Back, Core	Lift kettlebell to shoulder, flip grip at top. Repeat for 15 reps.
	(2) 20 V-Ups	Abs, Core, Hip Flexors	Lie back, lift legs and torso simultaneously. Repeat for 20 reps.
	(3) 20 Kettlebell Goblet Squats	Legs, Glutes, Core	Squat holding kettlebell close to chest. Repeat for 20 reps.
	(4) 250-meter run	Legs, Cardio, Core	Run 250 meters at a steady pace.
	Repeat 4 times with 1-minute rest between rounds:		
20	30 seconds Kettlebell Swing	Lower Body, Core, Shoulders	Swing kettlebell between legs, thrust hips forward, raise kettlebell to shoulder height. Repeat for 30 seconds.
	30 seconds Push-Ups	Chest, Triceps, Core	Lower body to ground, push up with arms. Repeat for 30 seconds.
	30 seconds Kettlebell Goblet Squats	Legs, Glutes, Core	Squat holding kettlebell close to chest. Repeat for 30 seconds.
	30 seconds Mountain Climbers	Cardio, Core, Legs	Run in place in plank position, drive knees to chest. Repeat for 30 seconds.

Workout No.	Workout (Kettlebell & Body-Weight Workouts)	Main Muscle Groups	Instructions
	3 Rounds for time:		
21	(1) 10 Kettlebell Deadlifts	Lower Back, Hamstrings, Glutes	Lift kettlebell from ground, keep back straight. Repeat for 10 reps.
	(2) 15 Push-Ups	Chest, Triceps, Core	Lower body to ground, push up with arms. Repeat for 15 reps.
	(3) 20 Kettlebell Goblet Squats	Legs, Glutes, Core	Squat holding kettlebell close to chest. Repeat for 20 reps.
	(4) 200-meter run	Legs, Cardio, Core	Run 200 meters at a steady pace.
	Repeat 4 times with 1-minute rest between rounds:		
22	(1) 30 seconds Kettlebell Swing	Lower Body, Core, Shoulders	Swing kettlebell between legs, thrust hips forward, raise kettlebell to shoulder height. Repeat for 30 seconds.
	(2) 30 seconds Mountain Climbers	Cardio, Core, Legs	Run in place in plank position, drive knees to chest. Repeat for 30 seconds.
	(3) 30 seconds Kettlebell Thrusters	Shoulders, Legs, Core	Squat to overhead press in one fluid motion. Repeat for 30 seconds.
	(4) 30 seconds Jumping Jacks	Cardio, Legs, Core	Jump to spread legs and clap hands overhead. Repeat for 30 seconds.
	3 Rounds for time:		
23	(1) 15 Kettlebell Clean and Press	Shoulders, Arms, Core	Clean kettlebell to shoulder, press overhead. Alternate arms. Complete 15 reps each arm.
	(2) 20 Air Squats	Legs, Glutes, Core	Stand, bend knees to lower body. Repeat for 20 reps.
	(3) 15 Kettlebell Bent Over Rows	Back, Shoulders, Arms	Hinge forward, row kettlebell to hip. Repeat for 15 reps each side.
	(4) 400-meter run	Legs, Cardio, Core	Run 400 meters at a steady pace.
	Repeat 5 times:		
24	(1) 40 seconds Kettlebell Snatch	Shoulders, Back, Core	Lift kettlebell overhead in one motion, lock arm. Alternate arms. Repeat for 40 seconds.
	(2) 20 seconds Rest		Rest for 20 seconds.
	(3) 40 seconds Burpees	Full Body, Core, Legs	Jump, squat down, kick back into push-up, return up. Repeat for 40 seconds.
	(4) 20 seconds Rest		Rest for 20 seconds.
	4 Rounds for time:		
25	(1) 20 Kettlebell Swings	Lower Body, Core, Shoulders	Swing kettlebell between legs, thrust hips forward. Repeat for 20 reps.
	(2) 20 Lunges	Legs, Glutes, Core	Step forward, lower hips to drop knee to ground. Repeat for 20 reps.
	(3) 15 Kettlebell Shoulder Press	Shoulders, Arms, Core	Press kettlebell overhead from shoulder level. Repeat for 15 reps each side.
	(4) 200-meter run	Legs, Cardio, Core	Run 200 meters at a steady pace.

Workout No.		Workout (Kettlebell & Body-Weight Workouts)	Main Muscle Groups	Instructions
		Repeat 5 times:		
	(1)	45 seconds Kettlebell Around the Body	Core, Shoulders, Arms	Pass kettlebell around body, maintain core control. Repeat for 45 seconds.
26	(2)	15 seconds Rest		Rest for 15 seconds.
	(3)	45 seconds Jumping Jacks	Cardio, Legs, Core	Jump to spread legs and clap hands overhead. Repeat for 45 seconds.
	(4)	15 seconds Rest		Rest for 15 seconds.
		3 Rounds for time:		
	(1)	10 Kettlebell Snatches	Shoulders, Back, Core	Lift kettlebell overhead in one motion, lock arm. Alternate arms. Complete 10 reps each arm.
27	(2)	20 Push-Ups	Chest, Triceps, Core	Lower body to ground, push up with arms. Repeat for 20 reps.
	(3)	15 Kettlebell Deadlifts	Lower Back, Hamstrings, Glutes	Lift kettlebell from ground, keep back straight. Repeat for 15 reps.
	(4)	300-meter run	Legs, Cardio, Core	Run 300 meters at a steady pace.
		Repeat 8 times:		
	(1)	20 seconds Kettlebell Jump Swing	Legs, Core, Shoulders	Explosive swing with a jump at top of motion. Repeat for 20 seconds.
28	(2)	10 seconds Rest		Rest for 10 seconds.
	(3)	20 seconds High Knees	Legs, Cardio, Core	Run in place lifting knees high. Repeat for 20 seconds.
	(4)	10 seconds Rest		Rest for 10 seconds.
		4 Rounds for time:		
	(1)	15 Kettlebell Clean	Shoulders, Back, Core	Lift kettlebell to shoulder, flip grip at top. Repeat for 15 reps.
29	(2)	20 V-Ups	Abs, Core, Hip Flexors	Lie back, lift legs and torso simultaneously. Repeat for 20 reps.
	(3)	20 Kettlebell Goblet Squats	Legs, Glutes, Core	Squat holding kettlebell close to chest. Repeat for 20 reps.
	(4)	250-meter run	Legs, Cardio, Core	Run 250 meters at a steady pace.
		Repeat 4 times with 1-minute rest between rounds:		
	(1)	30 seconds Kettlebell Swing	Lower Body, Core, Shoulders	Swing kettlebell between legs, thrust hips forward, raise kettlebell to shoulder height. Repeat for 30 seconds.
30	(2)	30 seconds Push-Ups	Chest, Triceps, Core	Lower body to ground, push up with arms. Repeat for 30 seconds.
	(3)	30 seconds Kettlebell Goblet Squats	Legs, Glutes, Core	Squat holding kettlebell close to chest. Repeat for 30 seconds.
	(4)	30 seconds Mountain Climbers	Cardio, Core, Legs	Run in place in plank position, drive knees to chest. Repeat for 30 seconds.

Workout No.	Workout (Kettlebell & Body-Weight Workouts)	Main Muscle Groups	Instructions
	3 Rounds for time:		
	(1) 10 Kettlebell Deadlifts	Lower Back, Hamstrings, Glutes	Lift kettlebell from ground, keep back straight. Repeat for 10 reps.
31	(2) 15 Push-Ups	Chest, Triceps, Core	Lower body to ground, push up with arms. Repeat for 15 reps.
	(3) 20 Kettlebell Goblet Squats	Legs, Glutes, Core	Squat holding kettlebell close to chest. Repeat for 20 reps.
	(4) 200-meter run	Legs, Cardio, Core	Run 200 meters at a steady pace.
	Repeat 4 times with 1-minute rest between rounds:		
	(1) 30 seconds Kettlebell Swing	Lower Body, Core, Shoulders	Swing kettlebell between legs, thrust hips forward, raise kettlebell to shoulder height. Repeat for 30 seconds.
32	(2) 30 seconds Mountain Climbers	Cardio, Core, Legs	Run in place in plank position, drive knees to chest. Repeat for 30 seconds.
	(3) 30 seconds Kettlebell Thrusters	Shoulders, Legs, Core	Squat to overhead press in one fluid motion. Repeat for 30 seconds.
	(4) 30 seconds Jumping Jacks	Cardio, Legs, Core	Jump to spread legs and clap hands overhead. Repeat for 30 seconds.
	3 Rounds for time:		
	(1) 15 Kettlebell Clean and Press	Shoulders, Arms, Core	Clean kettlebell to shoulder, press overhead. Alternate arms. Complete 15 reps each arm.
33	(2) 20 Air Squats	Legs, Glutes, Core	Stand, bend knees to lower body. Repeat for 20 reps.
	(3) 15 Kettlebell Bent Over Rows	Back, Shoulders, Arms	Hinge forward, row kettlebell to hip. Repeat for 15 reps each side.
	(4) 400-meter run	Legs, Cardio, Core	Run 400 meters at a steady pace.
	Repeat 5 times:		
	(1) 40 seconds Kettlebell Snatch	Shoulders, Back, Core	Lift kettlebell overhead in one motion, lock arm. Alternate arms. Repeat for 40 seconds.
34	(2) 20 seconds Rest		Rest for 20 seconds.
	(3) 40 seconds Burpees	Full Body, Core, Legs	Jump, squat down, kick back into push-up, return up. Repeat for 40 seconds.
	(4) 20 seconds Rest		Rest for 20 seconds.
	4 Rounds for time:		
	(1) 20 Kettlebell Swings	Lower Body, Core, Shoulders	Swing kettlebell between legs, thrust hips forward. Repeat for 20 reps.
35	(2) 20 Lunges	Legs, Glutes, Core	Step forward, lower hips to drop knee to ground. Repeat for 20 reps.
	(3) 15 Kettlebell Shoulder Press	Shoulders, Arms, Core	Press kettlebell overhead from shoulder level. Repeat for 15 reps each side.
	(4) 200-meter run	Legs, Cardio, Core	Run 200 meters at a steady pace.

Workout No.		Workout (Kettlebell & Body-Weight Workouts)	Main Muscle Groups	Instructions
36		**Repeat 5 times:**		
	(1)	45 seconds Kettlebell Around the Body	Core, Shoulders, Arms	Pass kettlebell around body, maintain core control. Repeat for 45 seconds.
	(2)	15 seconds Rest		Rest for 15 seconds.
	(3)	45 seconds Jumping Jacks	Cardio, Legs, Core	Jump to spread legs and clap hands overhead. Repeat for 45 seconds.
	(4)	15 seconds Rest		Rest for 15 seconds.
37		**3 Rounds for time:**		
	(1)	10 Kettlebell Snatches	Shoulders, Back, Core	Lift kettlebell overhead in one motion, lock arm. Alternate arms. Complete 10 reps each arm.
	(2)	20 Push-Ups	Chest, Triceps, Core	Lower body to ground, push up with arms. Repeat for 20 reps.
	(3)	15 Kettlebell Deadlifts	Lower Back, Hamstrings, Glutes	Lift kettlebell from ground, keep back straight. Repeat for 15 reps.
	(4)	300-meter run	Legs, Cardio, Core	Run 300 meters at a steady pace.
38		**Repeat 8 times:**		
	(1)	20 seconds Kettlebell Jump Swing	Legs, Core, Shoulders	Explosive swing with a jump at top of motion. Repeat for 20 seconds.
	(2)	10 seconds Rest		Rest for 10 seconds.
	(3)	20 seconds High Knees	Legs, Cardio, Core	Run in place lifting knees high. Repeat for 20 seconds.
	(4)	10 seconds Rest		Rest for 10 seconds.
39		**4 Rounds for time:**		
	(1)	15 Kettlebell Clean	Shoulders, Back, Core	Lift kettlebell to shoulder, flip grip at top. Repeat for 15 reps.
	(2)	20 V-Ups	Abs, Core, Hip Flexors	Lie back, lift legs and torso simultaneously. Repeat for 20 reps.
	(3)	20 Kettlebell Goblet Squats	Legs, Glutes, Core	Squat holding kettlebell close to chest. Repeat for 20 reps.
	(4)	250-meter run	Legs, Cardio, Core	Run 250 meters at a steady pace.
40		**Repeat 4 times with 1-minute rest between rounds:**		
	(1)	30 seconds Kettlebell Swing	Lower Body, Core, Shoulders	Swing kettlebell between legs, thrust hips forward, raise kettlebell to shoulder height. Repeat for 30 seconds.
	(2)	30 seconds Push-Ups	Chest, Triceps, Core	Lower body to ground, push up with arms. Repeat for 30 seconds.
	(3)	30 seconds Kettlebell Goblet Squats	Legs, Glutes, Core	Squat holding kettlebell close to chest. Repeat for 30 seconds.
	(4)	30 seconds Mountain Climbers	Cardio, Core, Legs	Run in place in plank position, drive knees to chest. Repeat for 30 seconds.

Workout No.	Workout (Kettlebell & Body-Weight Workouts)	Main Muscle Groups	Instructions
	3 Rounds for time:		
	(1) 10 Kettlebell Deadlifts	Lower Back, Hamstrings, Glutes	Lift kettlebell from ground, keep back straight. Repeat for 10 reps.
41	(2) 15 Push-Ups	Chest, Triceps, Core	Lower body to ground, push up with arms. Repeat for 15 reps.
	(3) 20 Kettlebell Goblet Squats	Legs, Glutes, Core	Squat holding kettlebell close to chest. Repeat for 20 reps.
	(4) 200-meter run	Legs, Cardio, Core	Run 200 meters at a steady pace.
	Repeat 4 times with 1-minute rest between rounds:		
	(1) 30 seconds Kettlebell Swing	Lower Body, Core, Shoulders	Swing kettlebell between legs, thrust hips forward, raise kettlebell to shoulder height. Repeat for 30 seconds.
42	(2) 30 seconds Mountain Climbers	Cardio, Core, Legs	Run in place in plank position, drive knees to chest. Repeat for 30 seconds.
	(3) 30 seconds Kettlebell Thrusters	Shoulders, Legs, Core	Squat to overhead press in one fluid motion. Repeat for 30 seconds.
	(4) 30 seconds Jumping Jacks	Cardio, Legs, Core	Jump to spread legs and clap hands overhead. Repeat for 30 seconds.
	3 Rounds for time:		
	(1) 15 Kettlebell Clean and Press	Shoulders, Arms, Core	Clean kettlebell to shoulder, press overhead. Alternate arms. Complete 15 reps each arm.
43	(2) 20 Air Squats	Legs, Glutes, Core	Stand, bend knees to lower body. Repeat for 20 reps.
	(3) 15 Kettlebell Bent Over Rows	Back, Shoulders, Arms	Hinge forward, row kettlebell to hip. Repeat for 15 reps each side.
	(4) 400-meter run	Legs, Cardio, Core	Run 400 meters at a steady pace.
	Repeat 5 times:		
	(1) 40 seconds Kettlebell Snatch	Shoulders, Back, Core	Lift kettlebell overhead in one motion, lock arm. Alternate arms. Repeat for 40 seconds.
44	(2) 20 seconds Rest		Rest for 20 seconds.
	(3) 40 seconds Burpees	Full Body, Core, Legs	Jump, squat down, kick back into push-up, return up. Repeat for 40 seconds.
	(4) 20 seconds Rest		Rest for 20 seconds.
	4 Rounds for time:		
	(1) 20 Kettlebell Swings	Lower Body, Core, Shoulders	Swing kettlebell between legs, thrust hips forward. Repeat for 20 reps.
45	(2) 20 Lunges	Legs, Glutes, Core	Step forward, lower hips to drop knee to ground. Repeat for 20 reps.
	(3) 15 Kettlebell Shoulder Press	Shoulders, Arms, Core	Press kettlebell overhead from shoulder level. Repeat for 15 reps each side.
	(4) 200-meter run	Legs, Cardio, Core	Run 200 meters at a steady pace.

Workout No.		Workout (Kettlebell & Body-Weight Workouts)	Main Muscle Groups	Instructions
		Repeat 5 times:		
46	(1)	45 seconds Kettlebell Around the Body	Core, Shoulders, Arms	Pass kettlebell around body, maintain core control. Repeat for 45 seconds.
	(2)	15 seconds Rest		Rest for 15 seconds.
	(3)	45 seconds Jumping Jacks	Cardio, Legs, Core	Jump to spread legs and clap hands overhead. Repeat for 45 seconds.
	(4)	15 seconds Rest		Rest for 15 seconds.
		3 Rounds for time:		
47	(1)	10 Kettlebell Snatches	Shoulders, Back, Core	Lift kettlebell overhead in one motion, lock arm. Alternate arms. Complete 10 reps each arm.
	(2)	20 Push-Ups	Chest, Triceps, Core	Lower body to ground, push up with arms. Repeat for 20 reps.
	(3)	15 Kettlebell Deadlifts	Lower Back, Hamstrings, Glutes	Lift kettlebell from ground, keep back straight. Repeat for 15 reps.
	(4)	300-meter run	Legs, Cardio, Core	Run 300 meters at a steady pace.
		Repeat 8 times:		
48	(1)	20 seconds Kettlebell Jump Swing	Legs, Core, Shoulders	Explosive swing with a jump at top of motion. Repeat for 20 seconds.
	(2)	10 seconds Rest		Rest for 10 seconds.
	(3)	20 seconds High Knees	Legs, Cardio, Core	Run in place lifting knees high. Repeat for 20 seconds.
	(4)	10 seconds Rest		Rest for 10 seconds.
		4 Rounds for time:		
49	(1)	15 Kettlebell Clean	Shoulders, Back, Core	Lift kettlebell to shoulder, flip grip at top. Repeat for 15 reps.
	(2)	20 V-Ups	Abs, Core, Hip Flexors	Lie back, lift legs and torso simultaneously. Repeat for 20 reps.
	(3)	20 Kettlebell Goblet Squats	Legs, Glutes, Core	Squat holding kettlebell close to chest. Repeat for 20 reps.
	(4)	250-meter run	Legs, Cardio, Core	Run 250 meters at a steady pace.
		Repeat 4 times with 1-minute rest between rounds:		
50	(1)	30 seconds Kettlebell Swing	Lower Body, Core, Shoulders	Swing kettlebell between legs, thrust hips forward, raise kettlebell to shoulder height. Repeat for 30 seconds.
	(2)	30 seconds Push-Ups	Chest, Triceps, Core	Lower body to ground, push up with arms. Repeat for 30 seconds.
	(3)	30 seconds Kettlebell Goblet Squats	Legs, Glutes, Core	Squat holding kettlebell close to chest. Repeat for 30 seconds.
	(4)	30 seconds Mountain Climbers	Cardio, Core, Legs	Run in place in plank position, drive knees to chest. Repeat for 30 seconds.

Workout No.	Workout (Kettlebell & Body-Weight Workouts)	Main Muscle Groups	Instructions
	3 Rounds for time:		
	(1) 10 Kettlebell Deadlifts	Lower Back, Hamstrings, Glutes	Lift kettlebell from ground, keep back straight. Repeat for 10 reps.
51	(2) 15 Push-Ups	Chest, Triceps, Core	Lower body to ground, push up with arms. Repeat for 15 reps.
	(3) 20 Kettlebell Goblet Squats	Legs, Glutes, Core	Squat holding kettlebell close to chest. Repeat for 20 reps.
	(4) 200-meter run	Legs, Cardio, Core	Run 200 meters at a steady pace.
	Repeat 4 times with 1-minute rest between rounds:		
	(1) 30 seconds Kettlebell Swing	Lower Body, Core, Shoulders	Swing kettlebell between legs, thrust hips forward, raise kettlebell to shoulder height. Repeat for 30 seconds.
52	(2) 30 seconds Mountain Climbers	Cardio, Core, Legs	Run in place in plank position, drive knees to chest. Repeat for 30 seconds.
	(3) 30 seconds Kettlebell Thrusters	Shoulders, Legs, Core	Squat to overhead press in one fluid motion. Repeat for 30 seconds.
	(4) 30 seconds Jumping Jacks	Cardio, Legs, Core	Jump to spread legs and clap hands overhead. Repeat for 30 seconds.
	3 Rounds for time:		
	(1) 15 Kettlebell Clean and Press	Shoulders, Arms, Core	Clean kettlebell to shoulder, press overhead. Alternate arms. Complete 15 reps each arm.
53	(2) 20 Air Squats	Legs, Glutes, Core	Stand, bend knees to lower body. Repeat for 20 reps.
	(3) 15 Kettlebell Bent Over Rows	Back, Shoulders, Arms	Hinge forward, row kettlebell to hip. Repeat for 15 reps each side.
	(4) 400-meter run	Legs, Cardio, Core	Run 400 meters at a steady pace.
	Repeat 5 times:		
	(1) 40 seconds Kettlebell Snatch	Shoulders, Back, Core	Lift kettlebell overhead in one motion, lock arm. Alternate arms. Repeat for 40 seconds.
54	(2) 20 seconds Rest		Rest for 20 seconds.
	(3) 40 seconds Burpees	Full Body, Core, Legs	Jump, squat down, kick back into push-up, return up. Repeat for 40 seconds.
	(4) 20 seconds Rest		Rest for 20 seconds.
	4 Rounds for time:		
	(1) 20 Kettlebell Swings	Lower Body, Core, Shoulders	Swing kettlebell between legs, thrust hips forward. Repeat for 20 reps.
55	(2) 20 Lunges	Legs, Glutes, Core	Step forward, lower hips to drop knee to ground. Repeat for 20 reps.
	(3) 15 Kettlebell Shoulder Press	Shoulders, Arms, Core	Press kettlebell overhead from shoulder level. Repeat for 15 reps each side.
	(4) 200-meter run	Legs, Cardio, Core	Run 200 meters at a steady pace.

Workout No.	Workout (Kettlebell & Body-Weight Workouts)	Main Muscle Groups	Instructions
	Repeat 5 times:		
	(1) 45 seconds Kettlebell Around the Body	Core, Shoulders, Arms	Pass kettlebell around body, maintain core control. Repeat for 45 seconds.
56	(2) 15 seconds Rest		Rest for 15 seconds.
	(3) 45 seconds Jumping Jacks	Cardio, Legs, Core	Jump to spread legs and clap hands overhead. Repeat for 45 seconds.
	(4) 15 seconds Rest		Rest for 15 seconds.
	3 Rounds for time:		
	(1) 10 Kettlebell Snatches	Shoulders, Back, Core	Lift kettlebell overhead in one motion, lock arm. Alternate arms. Complete 10 reps each arm.
57	(2) 20 Push-Ups	Chest, Triceps, Core	Lower body to ground, push up with arms. Repeat for 20 reps.
	(3) 15 Kettlebell Deadlifts	Lower Back, Hamstrings, Glutes	Lift kettlebell from ground, keep back straight. Repeat for 15 reps.
	(4) 300-meter run	Legs, Cardio, Core	Run 300 meters at a steady pace.
	Repeat 8 times:		
	(1) 20 seconds Kettlebell Jump Swing	Legs, Core, Shoulders	Explosive swing with a jump at top of motion. Repeat for 20 seconds.
58	(2) 10 seconds Rest		Rest for 10 seconds.
	(3) 20 seconds High Knees	Legs, Cardio, Core	Run in place lifting knees high. Repeat for 20 seconds.
	(4) 10 seconds Rest		Rest for 10 seconds.
	4 Rounds for time:		
	(1) 15 Kettlebell Clean	Shoulders, Back, Core	Lift kettlebell to shoulder, flip grip at top. Repeat for 15 reps.
59	(2) 20 V-Ups	Abs, Core, Hip Flexors	Lie back, lift legs and torso simultaneously. Repeat for 20 reps.
	(3) 20 Kettlebell Goblet Squats	Legs, Glutes, Core	Squat holding kettlebell close to chest. Repeat for 20 reps.
	(4) 250-meter run	Legs, Cardio, Core	Run 250 meters at a steady pace.
	Repeat 4 times with 1-minute rest between rounds:		
	(1) 30 seconds Kettlebell Swing	Lower Body, Core, Shoulders	Swing kettlebell between legs, thrust hips forward, raise kettlebell to shoulder height. Repeat for 30 seconds.
60	(2) 30 seconds Push-Ups	Chest, Triceps, Core	Lower body to ground, push up with arms. Repeat for 30 seconds.
	(3) 30 seconds Kettlebell Goblet Squats	Legs, Glutes, Core	Squat holding kettlebell close to chest. Repeat for 30 seconds.
	(4) 30 seconds Mountain Climbers	Cardio, Core, Legs	Run in place in plank position, drive knees to chest. Repeat for 30 seconds.

Workout No.	Workout (Kettlebell & Body-Weight Workouts)	Main Muscle Groups	Instructions
	3 Rounds for time:		
61	(1) 10 Kettlebell Deadlifts	Lower Back, Hamstrings, Glutes	Lift kettlebell from ground, keep back straight. Repeat for 10 reps.
	(2) 15 Push-Ups	Chest, Triceps, Core	Lower body to ground, push up with arms. Repeat for 15 reps.
	(3) 20 Kettlebell Goblet Squats	Legs, Glutes, Core	Squat holding kettlebell close to chest. Repeat for 20 reps.
	(4) 200-meter run	Legs, Cardio, Core	Run 200 meters at a steady pace.
	Repeat 4 times with 1-minute rest between rounds:		
62	(1) 30 seconds Kettlebell Swing	Lower Body, Core, Shoulders	Swing kettlebell between legs, thrust hips forward, raise kettlebell to shoulder height. Repeat for 30 seconds.
	(2) 30 seconds Mountain Climbers	Cardio, Core, Legs	Run in place in plank position, drive knees to chest. Repeat for 30 seconds.
	(3) 30 seconds Kettlebell Thrusters	Shoulders, Legs, Core	Squat to overhead press in one fluid motion. Repeat for 30 seconds.
	(4) 30 seconds Jumping Jacks	Cardio, Legs, Core	Jump to spread legs and clap hands overhead. Repeat for 30 seconds.
	3 Rounds for time:		
63	(1) 15 Kettlebell Clean and Press	Shoulders, Arms, Core	Clean kettlebell to shoulder, press overhead. Alternate arms. Complete 15 reps each arm.
	(2) 20 Air Squats	Legs, Glutes, Core	Stand, bend knees to lower body. Repeat for 20 reps.
	(3) 15 Kettlebell Bent Over Rows	Back, Shoulders, Arms	Hinge forward, row kettlebell to hip. Repeat for 15 reps each side.
	(4) 400-meter run	Legs, Cardio, Core	Run 400 meters at a steady pace.
	Repeat 5 times:		
64	(1) 40 seconds Kettlebell Snatch	Shoulders, Back, Core	Lift kettlebell overhead in one motion, lock arm. Alternate arms. Repeat for 40 seconds.
	(2) 20 seconds Rest		Rest for 20 seconds.
	(3) 40 seconds Burpees	Full Body, Core, Legs	Jump, squat down, kick back into push-up, return up. Repeat for 40 seconds.
	(4) 20 seconds Rest		Rest for 20 seconds.
	4 Rounds for time:		
65	(1) 20 Kettlebell Swings	Lower Body, Core, Shoulders	Swing kettlebell between legs, thrust hips forward. Repeat for 20 reps.
	(2) 20 Lunges	Legs, Glutes, Core	Step forward, lower hips to drop knee to ground. Repeat for 20 reps.
	(3) 15 Kettlebell Shoulder Press	Shoulders, Arms, Core	Press kettlebell overhead from shoulder level. Repeat for 15 reps each side.
	(4) 200-meter run	Legs, Cardio, Core	Run 200 meters at a steady pace.

Workout No.		Workout (Kettlebell & Body-Weight Workouts)	Main Muscle Groups	Instructions
66		**Repeat 5 times:**		
	(1)	45 seconds Kettlebell Around the Body	Core, Shoulders, Arms	Pass kettlebell around body, maintain core control. Repeat for 45 seconds.
	(2)	15 seconds Rest		Rest for 15 seconds.
	(3)	45 seconds Jumping Jacks	Cardio, Legs, Core	Jump to spread legs and clap hands overhead. Repeat for 45 seconds.
	(4)	15 seconds Rest		Rest for 15 seconds.
67		**3 Rounds for time:**		
	(1)	10 Kettlebell Snatches	Shoulders, Back, Core	Lift kettlebell overhead in one motion, lock arm. Alternate arms. Complete 10 reps each arm.
	(2)	20 Push-Ups	Chest, Triceps, Core	Lower body to ground, push up with arms. Repeat for 20 reps.
	(3)	15 Kettlebell Deadlifts	Lower Back, Hamstrings, Glutes	Lift kettlebell from ground, keep back straight. Repeat for 15 reps.
	(4)	300-meter run	Legs, Cardio, Core	Run 300 meters at a steady pace.
68		**Repeat 8 times:**		
	(1)	20 seconds Kettlebell Jump Swing	Legs, Core, Shoulders	Explosive swing with a jump at top of motion. Repeat for 20 seconds.
	(2)	10 seconds Rest		Rest for 10 seconds.
	(3)	20 seconds High Knees	Legs, Cardio, Core	Run in place lifting knees high. Repeat for 20 seconds.
	(4)	10 seconds Rest		Rest for 10 seconds.
69		**4 Rounds for time:**		
	(1)	15 Kettlebell Clean	Shoulders, Back, Core	Lift kettlebell to shoulder, flip grip at top. Repeat for 15 reps.
	(2)	20 V-Ups	Abs, Core, Hip Flexors	Lie back, lift legs and torso simultaneously. Repeat for 20 reps.
	(3)	20 Kettlebell Goblet Squats	Legs, Glutes, Core	Squat holding kettlebell close to chest. Repeat for 20 reps.
	(4)	250-meter run	Legs, Cardio, Core	Run 250 meters at a steady pace.
70		**Repeat 4 times with 1-minute rest between rounds:**		
	(1)	30 seconds Kettlebell Swing	Lower Body, Core, Shoulders	Swing kettlebell between legs, thrust hips forward, raise kettlebell to shoulder height. Repeat for 30 seconds.
	(2)	30 seconds Push-Ups	Chest, Triceps, Core	Lower body to ground, push up with arms. Repeat for 30 seconds.
	(3)	30 seconds Kettlebell Goblet Squats	Legs, Glutes, Core	Squat holding kettlebell close to chest. Repeat for 30 seconds.
	(4)	30 seconds Mountain Climbers	Cardio, Core, Legs	Run in place in plank position, drive knees to chest. Repeat for 30 seconds.

Workout No.	Workout (Kettlebell & Body-Weight Workouts)	Main Muscle Groups	Instructions
	3 Rounds for time:		
71	(1) 10 Kettlebell Deadlifts	Lower Back, Hamstrings, Glutes	Lift kettlebell from ground, keep back straight. Repeat for 10 reps.
	(2) 15 Push-Ups	Chest, Triceps, Core	Lower body to ground, push up with arms. Repeat for 15 reps.
	(3) 20 Kettlebell Goblet Squats	Legs, Glutes, Core	Squat holding kettlebell close to chest. Repeat for 20 reps.
	(4) 200-meter run	Legs, Cardio, Core	Run 200 meters at a steady pace.
	Repeat 4 times with 1-minute rest between rounds:		
72	(1) 30 seconds Kettlebell Swing	Lower Body, Core, Shoulders	Swing kettlebell between legs, thrust hips forward, raise kettlebell to shoulder height. Repeat for 30 seconds.
	(2) 30 seconds Mountain Climbers	Cardio, Core, Legs	Run in place in plank position, drive knees to chest. Repeat for 30 seconds.
	(3) 30 seconds Kettlebell Thrusters	Shoulders, Legs, Core	Squat to overhead press in one fluid motion. Repeat for 30 seconds.
	(4) 30 seconds Jumping Jacks	Cardio, Legs, Core	Jump to spread legs and clap hands overhead. Repeat for 30 seconds.
	3 Rounds for time:		
73	(1) 15 Kettlebell Clean and Press	Shoulders, Arms, Core	Clean kettlebell to shoulder, press overhead. Alternate arms. Complete 15 reps each arm.
	(2) 20 Air Squats	Legs, Glutes, Core	Stand, bend knees to lower body. Repeat for 20 reps.
	(3) 15 Kettlebell Bent Over Rows	Back, Shoulders, Arms	Hinge forward, row kettlebell to hip. Repeat for 15 reps each side.
	(4) 400-meter run	Legs, Cardio, Core	Run 400 meters at a steady pace.
	Repeat 5 times:		
74	(1) 40 seconds Kettlebell Snatch	Shoulders, Back, Core	Lift kettlebell overhead in one motion, lock arm. Alternate arms. Repeat for 40 seconds.
	(2) 20 seconds Rest		Rest for 20 seconds.
	(3) 40 seconds Burpees	Full Body, Core, Legs	Jump, squat down, kick back into push-up, return up. Repeat for 40 seconds.
	(4) 20 seconds Rest		Rest for 20 seconds.
	4 Rounds for time:		
75	(1) 20 Kettlebell Swings	Lower Body, Core, Shoulders	Swing kettlebell between legs, thrust hips forward. Repeat for 20 reps.
	(2) 20 Lunges	Legs, Glutes, Core	Step forward, lower hips to drop knee to ground. Repeat for 20 reps.
	(3) 15 Kettlebell Shoulder Press	Shoulders, Arms, Core	Press kettlebell overhead from shoulder level. Repeat for 15 reps each side.
	(4) 200-meter run	Legs, Cardio, Core	Run 200 meters at a steady pace.

Workout No.	Workout (Kettlebell & Body-Weight Workouts)	Main Muscle Groups	Instructions
	Repeat 5 times:		
	(1) 45 seconds Kettlebell Around the Body	Core, Shoulders, Arms	Pass kettlebell around body, maintain core control. Repeat for 45 seconds.
76	(2) 15 seconds Rest		Rest for 15 seconds.
	(3) 45 seconds Jumping Jacks	Cardio, Legs, Core	Jump to spread legs and clap hands overhead. Repeat for 45 seconds.
	(4) 15 seconds Rest		Rest for 15 seconds.
	3 Rounds for time:		
	(1) 10 Kettlebell Snatches	Shoulders, Back, Core	Lift kettlebell overhead in one motion, lock arm. Alternate arms. Complete 10 reps each arm.
77	(2) 20 Push-Ups	Chest, Triceps, Core	Lower body to ground, push up with arms. Repeat for 20 reps.
	(3) 15 Kettlebell Deadlifts	Lower Back, Hamstrings, Glutes	Lift kettlebell from ground, keep back straight. Repeat for 15 reps.
	(4) 300-meter run	Legs, Cardio, Core	Run 300 meters at a steady pace.
	Repeat 8 times:		
	(1) 20 seconds Kettlebell Jump Swing	Legs, Core, Shoulders	Explosive swing with a jump at top of motion. Repeat for 20 seconds.
78	(2) 10 seconds Rest		Rest for 10 seconds.
	(3) 20 seconds High Knees	Legs, Cardio, Core	Run in place lifting knees high. Repeat for 20 seconds.
	(4) 10 seconds Rest		Rest for 10 seconds.
	4 Rounds for time:		
	(1) 15 Kettlebell Clean	Shoulders, Back, Core	Lift kettlebell to shoulder, flip grip at top. Repeat for 15 reps.
79	(2) 20 V-Ups	Abs, Core, Hip Flexors	Lie back, lift legs and torso simultaneously. Repeat for 20 reps.
	(3) 20 Kettlebell Goblet Squats	Legs, Glutes, Core	Squat holding kettlebell close to chest. Repeat for 20 reps.
	(4) 250-meter run	Legs, Cardio, Core	Run 250 meters at a steady pace.
	Repeat 4 times with 1-minute rest between rounds:		
	(1) 30 seconds Kettlebell Swing	Lower Body, Core, Shoulders	Swing kettlebell between legs, thrust hips forward, raise kettlebell to shoulder height. Repeat for 30 seconds.
80	(2) 30 seconds Push-Ups	Chest, Triceps, Core	Lower body to ground, push up with arms. Repeat for 30 seconds.
	(3) 30 seconds Kettlebell Goblet Squats	Legs, Glutes, Core	Squat holding kettlebell close to chest. Repeat for 30 seconds.
	(4) 30 seconds Mountain Climbers	Cardio, Core, Legs	Run in place in plank position, drive knees to chest. Repeat for 30 seconds.

Workout No.	Workout (Kettlebell & Body-Weight Workouts)	Main Muscle Groups	Instructions
	4 Rounds for time:		
81	(1) 15 Kettlebell Deadlifts	Lower Back, Hamstrings, Glutes	Lift kettlebell from ground, keep back straight. Repeat for 15 reps.
	(2) 20 Push-Ups	Chest, Triceps, Core	Lower body to ground, push up with arms. Repeat for 20 reps.
	(3) 25 Kettlebell Goblet Squats	Legs, Glutes, Core	Squat holding kettlebell close to chest. Repeat for 25 reps.
	(4) 400-meter run	Legs, Cardio, Core	Run 400 meters at a steady pace.
	Repeat 4 times with 1-minute rest between rounds:		
82	(1) 30 seconds Kettlebell Swing	Lower Body, Core, Shoulders	Swing kettlebell between legs, thrust hips forward, raise kettlebell to shoulder height. Repeat for 30 seconds.
	(2) 30 seconds Mountain Climbers	Cardio, Core, Legs	Run in place in plank position, drive knees to chest. Repeat for 30 seconds.
	(3) 30 seconds Kettlebell Thrusters	Shoulders, Legs, Core	Squat to overhead press in one fluid motion. Repeat for 30 seconds.
	(4) 30 seconds Jumping Jacks	Cardio, Legs, Core	Jump to spread legs and clap hands overhead. Repeat for 30 seconds.
	3 Rounds for time:		
83	(1) 12 Kettlebell Clean and Press	Shoulders, Arms, Core	Clean kettlebell to shoulder, press overhead. Alternate arms. Complete 12 reps each arm.
	(2) 20 Air Squats	Legs, Glutes, Core	Stand, bend knees to lower body. Repeat for 20 reps.
	(3) 15 Kettlebell Bent Over Rows	Back, Shoulders, Arms	Hinge forward, row kettlebell to hip. Repeat for 15 reps each side.
	(4) 500-meter run	Legs, Cardio, Core	Run 500 meters at a steady pace.
	Repeat 5 times:		
84	(1) 40 seconds Kettlebell Snatch	Shoulders, Back, Core	Lift kettlebell overhead in one motion, lock arm. Alternate arms. Repeat for 40 seconds.
	(2) 20 seconds Rest		Rest for 20 seconds.
	(3) 40 seconds Burpees	Full Body, Core, Legs	Jump, squat down, kick back into push-up, return up. Repeat for 40 seconds.
	(4) 20 seconds Rest		Rest for 20 seconds.
	4 Rounds for time:		
85	(1) 20 Kettlebell Swings	Lower Body, Core, Shoulders	Swing kettlebell between legs, thrust hips forward. Repeat for 20 reps.
	(2) 20 Lunges	Legs, Glutes, Core	Step forward, lower hips to drop knee to ground. Repeat for 20 reps.
	(3) 15 Kettlebell Shoulder Press	Shoulders, Arms, Core	Press kettlebell overhead from shoulder level. Repeat for 15 reps each side
	(4) 300-meter run	Legs, Cardio, Core	Run 300 meters at a steady pace.

Workout No.	Workout (Kettlebell & Body-Weight Workouts)	Main Muscle Groups	Instructions
	Repeat 5 times:		
86	(1) 45 seconds Kettlebell Around the Body	Core, Shoulders, Arms	Pass kettlebell around body, maintain core control. Repeat for 45 seconds.
	(2) 15 seconds Rest		Rest for 15 seconds.
	(3) 45 seconds Jumping Jacks	Cardio, Legs, Core	Jump to spread legs and clap hands overhead. Repeat for 45 seconds.
	(4) 15 seconds Rest		Rest for 15 seconds.
	3 Rounds for time:		
87	(1) 10 Kettlebell Snatches	Shoulders, Back, Core	Lift kettlebell overhead in one motion, lock arm. Alternate arms. Complete 10 reps each arm.
	(2) 20 Push-Ups	Chest, Triceps, Core	Lower body to ground, push up with arms. Repeat for 20 reps.
	(3) 15 Kettlebell Deadlifts	Lower Back, Hamstrings, Glutes	Lift kettlebell from ground, keep back straight. Repeat for 15 reps.
	(4) 300-meter run	Legs, Cardio, Core	Run 300 meters at a steady pace.
	Repeat 8 times:		
88	(1) 20 seconds Kettlebell Jump Swing	Legs, Core, Shoulders	Explosive swing with a jump at top of motion. Repeat for 20 seconds.
	(2) 10 seconds Rest		Rest for 10 seconds.
	(3) 20 seconds High Knees	Legs, Cardio, Core	Run in place lifting knees high. Repeat for 20 seconds.
	(4) 10 seconds Rest		Rest for 10 seconds.
	4 Rounds for time:		
89	(1) 15 Kettlebell Clean	Shoulders, Back, Core	Lift kettlebell to shoulder, flip grip at top. Repeat for 15 reps.
	(2) 20 V-Ups	Abs, Core, Hip Flexors	Lie back, lift legs and torso simultaneously. Repeat for 20 reps.
	(3) 20 Kettlebell Goblet Squats	Legs, Glutes, Core	Squat holding kettlebell close to chest. Repeat for 20 reps.
	(4) 250-meter run	Legs, Cardio, Core	Run 250 meters at a steady pace.
	Repeat 4 times with 1-minute rest between rounds:		
90	(1) 30 seconds Kettlebell Swing	Lower Body, Core, Shoulders	Swing kettlebell between legs, thrust hips forward, raise kettlebell to shoulder height. Repeat for 30 seconds.
	(2) 30 seconds Push-Ups	Chest, Triceps, Core	Lower body to ground, push up with arms. Repeat for 30 seconds.
	(3) 30 seconds Kettlebell Goblet Squats	Legs, Glutes, Core	Squat holding kettlebell close to chest. Repeat for 30 seconds.
	(4) 30 seconds Mountain Climbers	Cardio, Core, Legs	Run in place in plank position, drive knees to chest. Repeat for 30 seconds.

Workout No.	Workout (Kettlebell & Body-Weight Workouts)	Main Muscle Groups	Instructions
	4 Rounds for time:		
91	(1) 15 Kettlebell Deadlifts	Lower Back, Hamstrings, Glutes	Lift kettlebell from ground, keep back straight. Repeat for 15 reps.
	(2) 20 Push-Ups	Chest, Triceps, Core	Lower body to ground, push up with arms. Repeat for 20 reps.
	(3) 25 Kettlebell Goblet Squats	Legs, Glutes, Core	Squat holding kettlebell close to chest. Repeat for 25 reps.
	(4) 400-meter run	Legs, Cardio, Core	Run 400 meters at a steady pace.
	Repeat 4 times with 1-minute rest between rounds:		
92	(1) 30 seconds Kettlebell Swing	Lower Body, Core, Shoulders	Swing kettlebell between legs, thrust hips forward, raise kettlebell to shoulder height. Repeat for 30 seconds.
	(2) 30 seconds Mountain Climbers	Cardio, Core, Legs	Run in place in plank position, drive knees to chest. Repeat for 30 seconds.
	(3) 30 seconds Kettlebell Thrusters	Shoulders, Legs, Core	Squat to overhead press in one fluid motion. Repeat for 30 seconds.
	(4) 30 seconds Jumping Jacks	Cardio, Legs, Core	Jump to spread legs and clap hands overhead. Repeat for 30 seconds.
	3 Rounds for time:		
93	(1) 12 Kettlebell Clean and Press	Shoulders, Arms, Core	Clean kettlebell to shoulder, press overhead. Alternate arms. Complete 12 reps each arm.
	(2) 20 Air Squats	Legs, Glutes, Core	Stand, bend knees to lower body. Repeat for 20 reps.
	(3) 15 Kettlebell Bent Over Rows	Back, Shoulders, Arms	Hinge forward, row kettlebell to hip. Repeat for 15 reps each side.
	(4) 500-meter run	Legs, Cardio, Core	Run 500 meters at a steady pace.
	Repeat 5 times:		
94	(1) 40 seconds Kettlebell Snatch	Shoulders, Back, Core	Lift kettlebell overhead in one motion, lock arm. Alternate arms. Repeat for 40 seconds.
	(2) 20 seconds Rest		Rest for 20 seconds.
	(3) 40 seconds Burpees	Full Body, Core, Legs	Jump, squat down, kick back into push-up, return up. Repeat for 40 seconds.
	(4) 20 seconds Rest		Rest for 20 seconds.
	4 Rounds for time:		
95	(1) 20 Kettlebell Swings	Lower Body, Core, Shoulders	Swing kettlebell between legs, thrust hips forward. Repeat for 20 reps.
	(2) 20 Lunges	Legs, Glutes, Core	Step forward, lower hips to drop knee to ground. Repeat for 20 reps.
	(3) 15 Kettlebell Shoulder Press	Shoulders, Arms, Core	Press kettlebell overhead from shoulder level. Repeat for 15 reps each side.
	(4) 300-meter run	Legs, Cardio, Core	Run 300 meters at a steady pace.

Workout No.	Workout (Kettlebell & Body-Weight Workouts)		Main Muscle Groups	Instructions
	Repeat 5 times:			
96	(1)	45 seconds Kettlebell Around the Body	Core, Shoulders, Arms	Pass kettlebell around body, maintain core control. Repeat for 45 seconds.
	(2)	15 seconds Rest		Rest for 15 seconds.
	(3)	45 seconds Jumping Jacks	Cardio, Legs, Core	Jump to spread legs and clap hands overhead. Repeat for 45 seconds.
	(4)	15 seconds Rest		Rest for 15 seconds.
	3 Rounds for time:			
97	(1)	10 Kettlebell Snatches	Shoulders, Back, Core	Lift kettlebell overhead in one motion, lock arm. Alternate arms. Complete 10 reps each arm.
	(2)	20 Push-Ups	Chest, Triceps, Core	Lower body to ground, push up with arms. Repeat for 20 reps.
	(3)	15 Kettlebell Deadlifts	Lower Back, Hamstrings, Glutes	Lift kettlebell from ground, keep back straight. Repeat for 15 reps.
	(4)	300-meter run	Legs, Cardio, Core	Run 300 meters at a steady pace.
	Repeat 8 times:			
98	(1)	20 seconds Kettlebell Jump Swing	Legs, Core, Shoulders	Explosive swing with a jump at top of motion. Repeat for 20 seconds.
	(2)	10 seconds Rest		Rest for 10 seconds.
	(3)	20 seconds High Knees	Legs, Cardio, Core	Run in place lifting knees high. Repeat for 20 seconds.
	(4)	10 seconds Rest		Rest for 10 seconds.
	4 Rounds for time:			
99	(1)	15 Kettlebell Clean	Shoulders, Back, Core	Lift kettlebell to shoulder, flip grip at top. Repeat for 15 reps.
	(2)	20 V-Ups	Abs, Core, Hip Flexors	Lie back, lift legs and torso simultaneously. Repeat for 20 reps.
	(3)	20 Kettlebell Goblet Squats	Legs, Glutes, Core	Squat holding kettlebell close to chest. Repeat for 20 reps.
	(4)	250-meter run	Legs, Cardio, Core	Run 250 meters at a steady pace.
	Repeat 4 times with 1-minute rest between rounds:			
100	(1)	30 seconds Kettlebell Swing	Lower Body, Core, Shoulders	Swing kettlebell between legs, thrust hips forward, raise kettlebell to shoulder height. Repeat for 30 seconds.
	(2)	30 seconds Push-Ups	Chest, Triceps, Core	Lower body to ground, push up with arms. Repeat for 30 seconds.
	(3)	30 seconds Kettlebell Goblet Squats	Legs, Glutes, Core	Squat holding kettlebell close to chest. Repeat for 30 seconds.
	(4)	30 seconds Mountain Climbers	Cardio, Core, Legs	Run in place in plank position, drive knees to chest. Repeat for 30 seconds.

Workout No.	Workout (Kettlebell & Body-Weight Workouts)	Main Muscle Groups	Instructions
	4 Rounds for time:		
	(1) 15 Kettlebell Deadlifts	Lower Back, Hamstrings, Glutes	Lift kettlebell from ground, keep back straight. Repeat for 15 reps.
101	(2) 20 Push-Ups	Chest, Triceps, Core	Lower body to ground, push up with arms. Repeat for 20 reps.
	(3) 25 Kettlebell Goblet Squats	Legs, Glutes, Core	Squat holding kettlebell close to chest. Repeat for 25 reps.
	(4) 400-meter run	Legs, Cardio, Core	Run 400 meters at a steady pace.
	Repeat 4 times with 1-minute rest between rounds:		
	(1) 30 seconds Kettlebell Swing	Lower Body, Core, Shoulders	Swing kettlebell between legs, thrust hips forward, raise kettlebell to shoulder height. Repeat for 30 seconds.
102	(2) 30 seconds Mountain Climbers	Cardio, Core, Legs	Run in place in plank position, drive knees to chest. Repeat for 30 seconds.
	(3) 30 seconds Kettlebell Thrusters	Shoulders, Legs, Core	Squat to overhead press in one fluid motion. Repeat for 30 seconds.
	(4) 30 seconds Jumping Jacks	Cardio, Legs, Core	Jump to spread legs and clap hands overhead. Repeat for 30 seconds.
	3 Rounds for time:		
	(1) 12 Kettlebell Clean and Press	Shoulders, Arms, Core	Clean kettlebell to shoulder, press overhead. Alternate arms. Complete 12 reps each arm.
103	(2) 20 Air Squats	Legs, Glutes, Core	Stand, bend knees to lower body. Repeat for 20 reps.
	(3) 15 Kettlebell Bent Over Rows	Back, Shoulders, Arms	Hinge forward, row kettlebell to hip. Repeat for 15 reps each side.
	(4) 500-meter run	Legs, Cardio, Core	Run 500 meters at a steady pace.
	Repeat 5 times:		
	(1) 40 seconds Kettlebell Snatch	Shoulders, Back, Core	Lift kettlebell overhead in one motion, lock arm. Alternate arms. Repeat for 40 seconds.
104	(2) 20 seconds Rest		Rest for 20 seconds.
	(3) 40 seconds Burpees	Full Body, Core, Legs	Jump, squat down, kick back into push-up, return up. Repeat for 40 seconds.
	(4) 20 seconds Rest		Rest for 20 seconds.
	4 Rounds for time:		
	(1) 20 Kettlebell Swings	Lower Body, Core, Shoulders	Swing kettlebell between legs, thrust hips forward. Repeat for 20 reps.
105	(2) 20 Lunges	Legs, Glutes, Core	Step forward, lower hips to drop knee to ground. Repeat for 20 reps.
	(3) 15 Kettlebell Shoulder Press	Shoulders, Arms, Core	Press kettlebell overhead from shoulder level. Repeat for 15 reps each side.
	(4) 300-meter run	Legs, Cardio, Core	Run 300 meters at a steady pace.

Workout No.	Workout (Kettlebell & Body-Weight Workouts)	Main Muscle Groups	Instructions
	Repeat 5 times:		
	(1) 45 seconds Kettlebell Around the Body	Core, Shoulders, Arms	Pass kettlebell around body, maintain core control. Repeat for 45 seconds.
106	(2) 15 seconds Rest		Rest for 15 seconds.
	(3) 45 seconds Jumping Jacks	Cardio, Legs, Core	Jump to spread legs and clap hands overhead. Repeat for 45 seconds.
	(4) 15 seconds Rest		Rest for 15 seconds.
	3 Rounds for time:		
	(1) 10 Kettlebell Snatches	Shoulders, Back, Core	Lift kettlebell overhead in one motion, lock arm. Alternate arms. Complete 10 reps each arm.
107	(2) 20 Push-Ups	Chest, Triceps, Core	Lower body to ground, push up with arms. Repeat for 20 reps.
	(3) 15 Kettlebell Deadlifts	Lower Back, Hamstrings, Glutes	Lift kettlebell from ground, keep back straight. Repeat for 15 reps.
	(4) 300-meter run	Legs, Cardio, Core	Run 300 meters at a steady pace.
	Repeat 8 times:		
	(1) 20 seconds Kettlebell Jump Swing	Legs, Core, Shoulders	Explosive swing with a jump at top of motion. Repeat for 20 seconds.
108	(2) 10 seconds Rest		Rest for 10 seconds.
	(3) 20 seconds High Knees	Legs, Cardio, Core	Run in place lifting knees high. Repeat for 20 seconds.
	(4) 10 seconds Rest		Rest for 10 seconds.
	4 Rounds for time:		
	(1) 15 Kettlebell Clean	Shoulders, Back, Core	Lift kettlebell to shoulder, flip grip at top. Repeat for 15 reps.
109	(2) 20 V-Ups	Abs, Core, Hip Flexors	Lie back, lift legs and torso simultaneously. Repeat for 20 reps.
	(3) 20 Kettlebell Goblet Squats	Legs, Glutes, Core	Squat holding kettlebell close to chest. Repeat for 20 reps.
	(4) 250-meter run	Legs, Cardio, Core	Run 250 meters at a steady pace.
	Repeat 4 times with 1-minute rest between rounds:		
	(1) 30 seconds Kettlebell Swing	Lower Body, Core, Shoulders	Swing kettlebell between legs, thrust hips forward, raise kettlebell to shoulder height. Repeat for 30 seconds.
110	(2) 30 seconds Push-Ups	Chest, Triceps, Core	Lower body to ground, push up with arms. Repeat for 30 seconds.
	(3) 30 seconds Kettlebell Goblet Squats	Legs, Glutes, Core	Squat holding kettlebell close to chest. Repeat for 30 seconds.
	(4) 30 seconds Mountain Climbers	Cardio, Core, Legs	Run in place in plank position, drive knees to chest. Repeat for 30 seconds.

Workout No.	Workout (Kettlebell & Body-Weight Workouts)	Main Muscle Groups	Instructions
	4 Rounds for time:		
	(1) 15 Kettlebell Swings	Lower Body, Core, Shoulders	Swing kettlebell between legs, thrust hips forward. Repeat for 15 reps.
111	(2) 20 Air Squats	Legs, Glutes, Core	Stand, bend knees to lower body. Repeat for 20 reps.
	(3) 12 Kettlebell Clean and Press	Shoulders, Arms, Core	Clean kettlebell to shoulder, press overhead. Repeat for 12 reps each arm.
	(4) 400-meter run	Legs, Cardio, Core	Run 400 meters at a steady pace.
	Repeat 4 times with 1-minute rest between rounds:		
	(1) 30 seconds Kettlebell Snatch	Shoulders, Back, Core	Lift kettlebell overhead in one motion. Alternate arms. Repeat for 30 seconds.
112	(2) 30 seconds Mountain Climbers	Cardio, Core, Legs	Run in place in plank position, drive knees to chest. Repeat for 30 seconds.
	(3) 30 seconds Kettlebell Thrusters	Shoulders, Legs, Core	Squat to overhead press in one fluid motion. Repeat for 30 seconds.
	(4) 30 seconds Jumping Jacks	Cardio, Legs, Core	Jump to spread legs and clap hands overhead. Repeat for 30 seconds.
	3 Rounds for time:		
	(1) 12 Kettlebell Deadlifts	Lower Back, Hamstrings, Glutes	Lift kettlebell from ground, keep back straight. Repeat for 12 reps.
113	(2) 20 Push-Ups	Chest, Triceps, Core	Lower body to ground, push up with arms. Repeat for 20 reps.
	(3) 15 Kettlebell Bent Over Rows	Back, Shoulders, Arms	Hinge forward, row kettlebell to hip. Repeat for 15 reps each side.
	(4) 500-meter run	Legs, Cardio, Core	Run 500 meters at a steady pace.
	Repeat 5 times:		
	(1) 40 seconds Kettlebell Around the Body	Core, Shoulders, Arms	Pass kettlebell around body, maintain core control. Repeat for 40 seconds.
114	(2) 20 seconds Rest		Rest for 20 seconds.
	(3) 40 seconds Burpees	Full Body, Core, Legs	Jump, squat down, kick back into push-up, return up. Repeat for 40 seconds.
	(4) 20 seconds Rest		Rest for 20 seconds.
	4 Rounds for time:		
	(1) 20 Kettlebell Snatches	Shoulders, Back, Core	Lift kettlebell overhead in one motion. Alternate arms. Repeat for 20 reps each arm.
115	(2) 20 Lunges	Legs, Glutes, Core	Step forward, lower hips to drop knee to ground. Repeat for 20 reps.
	(3) 20 Kettlebell Goblet Squats	Legs, Glutes, Core	Squat holding kettlebell close to chest. Repeat for 20 reps.
	(4) 300-meter run	Legs, Cardio, Core	Run 300 meters at a steady pace.

Workout No.	Workout (Kettlebell & Body-Weight Workouts)	Main Muscle Groups	Instructions
	Repeat 5 times:		
116	(1) 45 seconds Kettlebell Jump Swing	Legs, Core, Shoulders	Explosive swing with a jump at top of motion. Repeat for 45 seconds.
	(2) 15 seconds Rest		Rest for 15 seconds.
	(3) 45 seconds Jumping Jacks	Cardio, Legs, Core	Jump to spread legs and clap hands overhead. Repeat for 45 seconds.
	(4) 15 seconds Rest		Rest for 15 seconds.
	3 Rounds for time:		
117	(1) 10 Kettlebell Clean and Press	Shoulders, Arms, Core	Clean kettlebell to shoulder, press overhead. Repeat for 10 reps each arm.
	(2) 20 Push-Ups	Chest, Triceps, Core	Lower body to ground, push up with arms. Repeat for 20 reps.
	(3) 15 Kettlebell Deadlifts	Lower Back, Hamstrings, Glutes	Lift kettlebell from ground, keep back straight. Repeat for 15 reps.
	(4) 300-meter run	Legs, Cardio, Core	Run 300 meters at a steady pace.
	Repeat 8 times:		
118	(1) 20 seconds Kettlebell Atlas Swing	Shoulders, Back, Core	Swing kettlebell up, catch at chest level. Repeat for 20 seconds.
	(2) 10 seconds Rest		Rest for 10 seconds.
	(3) 20 seconds High Knees	Legs, Cardio, Core	Run in place lifting knees high. Repeat for 20 seconds.
	(4) 10 seconds Rest		Rest for 10 seconds.
	4 Rounds for time:		
119	(1) 15 Kettlebell Clean	Shoulders, Back, Core	Lift kettlebell to shoulder, flip grip at top. Repeat for 15 reps.
	(2) 20 V-Ups	Abs, Core, Hip Flexors	Lie back, lift legs and torso simultaneously. Repeat for 20 reps.
	(3) 20 Kettlebell Goblet Squats	Legs, Glutes, Core	Squat holding kettlebell close to chest. Repeat for 20 reps.
	(4) 250-meter run	Legs, Cardio, Core	Run 250 meters at a steady pace.
	Repeat 4 times with 1-minute rest between rounds:		
120	(1) 30 seconds Kettlebell Swing	Lower Body, Core, Shoulders	Swing kettlebell between legs, thrust hips forward, raise kettlebell to shoulder height. Repeat for 30 seconds.
	(2) 30 seconds Push-Ups	Chest, Triceps, Core	Lower body to ground, push up with arms. Repeat for 30 seconds.
	(3) 30 seconds Kettlebell Goblet Squats	Legs, Glutes, Core	Squat holding kettlebell close to chest. Repeat for 30 seconds.
	(4) 30 seconds Mountain Climbers	Cardio, Core, Legs	Run in place in plank position, drive knees to chest. Repeat for 30 seconds.

Workout No.	Workout (Kettlebell & Body-Weight Workouts)	Main Muscle Groups	Instructions
	4 Rounds for time:		
	(1) 15 Kettlebell Swings	Lower Body, Core, Shoulders	Swing kettlebell between legs, thrust hips forward. Repeat for 15 reps.
121	(2) 20 Air Squats	Legs, Glutes, Core	Stand, bend knees to lower body. Repeat for 20 reps.
	(3) 12 Kettlebell Clean and Press	Shoulders, Arms, Core	Clean kettlebell to shoulder, press overhead. Repeat for 12 reps each arm.
	(4) 400-meter run	Legs, Cardio, Core	Run 400 meters at a steady pace.
	Repeat 4 times with 1-minute rest between rounds:		
	(1) 30 seconds Kettlebell Snatch	Shoulders, Back, Core	Lift kettlebell overhead in one motion. Alternate arms. Repeat for 30 seconds.
122	(2) 30 seconds Mountain Climbers	Cardio, Core, Legs	Run in place in plank position, drive knees to chest. Repeat for 30 seconds.
	(3) 30 seconds Kettlebell Thrusters	Shoulders, Legs, Core	Squat to overhead press in one fluid motion. Repeat for 30 seconds.
	(4) 30 seconds Jumping Jacks	Cardio, Legs, Core	Jump to spread legs and clap hands overhead. Repeat for 30 seconds.
	3 Rounds for time:		
	(1) 12 Kettlebell Deadlifts	Lower Back, Hamstrings, Glutes	Lift kettlebell from ground, keep back straight. Repeat for 12 reps.
123	(2) 20 Push-Ups	Chest, Triceps, Core	Lower body to ground, push up with arms. Repeat for 20 reps.
	(3) 15 Kettlebell Bent Over Rows	Back, Shoulders, Arms	Hinge forward, row kettlebell to hip. Repeat for 15 reps each side.
	(4) 500-meter run	Legs, Cardio, Core	Run 500 meters at a steady pace.
	Repeat 5 times:		
	(1) 40 seconds Kettlebell Around the Body	Core, Shoulders, Arms	Pass kettlebell around body, maintain core control. Repeat for 40 seconds.
124	(2) 20 seconds Rest		Rest for 20 seconds.
	(3) 40 seconds Burpees	Full Body, Core, Legs	Jump, squat down, kick back into push-up, return up. Repeat for 40 seconds.
	(4) 20 seconds Rest		Rest for 20 seconds.
	4 Rounds for time:		
	(1) 20 Kettlebell Snatches	Shoulders, Back, Core	Lift kettlebell overhead in one motion. Alternate arms. Repeat for 20 reps each arm.
125	(2) 20 Lunges	Legs, Glutes, Core	Step forward, lower hips to drop knee to ground. Repeat for 20 reps.
	(3) 20 Kettlebell Goblet Squats	Legs, Glutes, Core	Squat holding kettlebell close to chest. Repeat for 20 reps.
	(4) 300-meter run	Legs, Cardio, Core	Run 300 meters at a steady pace.

Workout No.		Workout (Kettlebell & Body-Weight Workouts)	Main Muscle Groups	Instructions
		Repeat 5 times:		
126	(1)	45 seconds Kettlebell Jump Swing	Legs, Core, Shoulders	Explosive swing with a jump at top of motion. Repeat for 45 seconds.
	(2)	15 seconds Rest		Rest for 15 seconds.
	(3)	45 seconds Jumping Jacks	Cardio, Legs, Core	Jump to spread legs and clap hands overhead. Repeat for 45 seconds.
	(4)	15 seconds Rest		Rest for 15 seconds.
		3 Rounds for time:		
127	(1)	10 Kettlebell Clean and Press	Shoulders, Arms, Core	Clean kettlebell to shoulder, press overhead. Repeat for 10 reps each arm.
	(2)	20 Push-Ups	Chest, Triceps, Core	Lower body to ground, push up with arms. Repeat for 20 reps.
	(3)	15 Kettlebell Deadlifts	Lower Back, Hamstrings, Glutes	Lift kettlebell from ground, keep back straight. Repeat for 15 reps.
	(4)	300-meter run	Legs, Cardio, Core	Run 300 meters at a steady pace.
		Repeat 8 times:		
128	(1)	20 seconds Kettlebell Atlas Swing	Shoulders, Back, Core	Swing kettlebell up, catch at chest level. Repeat for 20 seconds.
	(2)	10 seconds Rest		Rest for 10 seconds.
	(3)	20 seconds High Knees	Legs, Cardio, Core	Run in place lifting knees high. Repeat for 20 seconds.
	(4)	10 seconds Rest		Rest for 10 seconds.
		4 Rounds for time:		
129	(1)	15 Kettlebell Clean	Shoulders, Back, Core	Lift kettlebell to shoulder, flip grip at top. Repeat for 15 reps.
	(2)	20 V-Ups	Abs, Core, Hip Flexors	Lie back, lift legs and torso simultaneously. Repeat for 20 reps.
	(3)	20 Kettlebell Goblet Squats	Legs, Glutes, Core	Squat holding kettlebell close to chest. Repeat for 20 reps.
	(4)	250-meter run	Legs, Cardio, Core	Run 250 meters at a steady pace.
		Repeat 4 times with 1-minute rest between rounds:		
130	(1)	30 seconds Kettlebell Swing	Lower Body, Core, Shoulders	Swing kettlebell between legs, thrust hips forward, raise kettlebell to shoulder height. Repeat for 30 seconds.
	(2)	30 seconds Push-Ups	Chest, Triceps, Core	Lower body to ground, push up with arms. Repeat for 30 seconds.
	(3)	30 seconds Kettlebell Goblet Squats	Legs, Glutes, Core	Squat holding kettlebell close to chest. Repeat for 30 seconds.
	(4)	30 seconds Mountain Climbers	Cardio, Core, Legs	Run in place in plank position, drive knees to chest. Repeat for 30 seconds.

Workout No.	Workout (Kettlebell & Body-Weight Workouts)	Main Muscle Groups	Instructions
	4 Rounds for time:		
131	(1) 15 Kettlebell Swings	Lower Body, Core, Shoulders	Swing kettlebell between legs, thrust hips forward. Repeat for 15 reps.
	(2) 20 Air Squats	Legs, Glutes, Core	Stand, bend knees to lower body. Repeat for 20 reps.
	(3) 12 Kettlebell Clean and Press	Shoulders, Arms, Core	Clean kettlebell to shoulder, press overhead. Repeat for 12 reps each arm.
	(4) 400-meter run	Legs, Cardio, Core	Run 400 meters at a steady pace.
	Repeat 4 times with 1-minute rest between rounds:		
132	(1) 30 seconds Kettlebell Snatch	Shoulders, Back, Core	Lift kettlebell overhead in one motion. Alternate arms. Repeat for 30 seconds.
	(2) 30 seconds Mountain Climbers	Cardio, Core, Legs	Run in place in plank position, drive knees to chest. Repeat for 30 seconds.
	(3) 30 seconds Kettlebell Thrusters	Shoulders, Legs, Core	Squat to overhead press in one fluid motion. Repeat for 30 seconds.
	(4) 30 seconds Jumping Jacks	Cardio, Legs, Core	Jump to spread legs and clap hands overhead. Repeat for 30 seconds.
	3 Rounds for time:		
133	(1) 12 Kettlebell Deadlifts	Lower Back, Hamstrings, Glutes	Lift kettlebell from ground, keep back straight. Repeat for 12 reps.
	(2) 20 Push-Ups	Chest, Triceps, Core	Lower body to ground, push up with arms. Repeat for 20 reps.
	(3) 15 Kettlebell Bent Over Rows	Back, Shoulders, Arms	Hinge forward, row kettlebell to hip. Repeat for 15 reps each side.
	(4) 500-meter run	Legs, Cardio, Core	Run 500 meters at a steady pace.
	Repeat 5 times:		
134	(1) 40 seconds Kettlebell Around the Body	Core, Shoulders, Arms	Pass kettlebell around body, maintain core control. Repeat for 40 seconds.
	(2) 20 seconds Rest		Rest for 20 seconds.
	(3) 40 seconds Burpees	Full Body, Core, Legs	Jump, squat down, kick back into push-up, return up. Repeat for 40 seconds.
	(4) 20 seconds Rest		Rest for 20 seconds.
	4 Rounds for time:		
135	(1) 20 Kettlebell Snatches	Shoulders, Back, Core	Lift kettlebell overhead in one motion. Alternate arms. Repeat for 20 reps each arm.
	(2) 20 Lunges	Legs, Glutes, Core	Step forward, lower hips to drop knee to ground. Repeat for 20 reps.
	(3) 20 Kettlebell Goblet Squats	Legs, Glutes, Core	Squat holding kettlebell close to chest. Repeat for 20 reps.
	(4) 300-meter run	Legs, Cardio, Core	Run 300 meters at a steady pace.

Workout No.	Workout (Kettlebell & Body-Weight Workouts)	Main Muscle Groups	Instructions
	Repeat 5 times:		
	(1) 45 seconds Kettlebell Jump Swing	Legs, Core, Shoulders	Explosive swing with a jump at top of motion. Repeat for 45 seconds.
136	(2) 15 seconds Rest		Rest for 15 seconds.
	(3) 45 seconds Jumping Jacks	Cardio, Legs, Core	Jump to spread legs and clap hands overhead. Repeat for 45 seconds.
	(4) 15 seconds Rest		Rest for 15 seconds.
	3 Rounds for time:		
	(1) 10 Kettlebell Clean and Press	Shoulders, Arms, Core	Clean kettlebell to shoulder, press overhead. Repeat for 10 reps each arm.
137	(2) 20 Push-Ups	Chest, Triceps, Core	Lower body to ground, push up with arms. Repeat for 20 reps.
	(3) 15 Kettlebell Deadlifts	Lower Back, Hamstrings, Glutes	Lift kettlebell from ground, keep back straight. Repeat for 15 reps.
	(4) 300-meter run	Legs, Cardio, Core	Run 300 meters at a steady pace.
	Repeat 8 times:		
	(1) 20 seconds Kettlebell Atlas Swing	Shoulders, Back, Core	Swing kettlebell up, catch at chest level. Repeat for 20 seconds.
138	(2) 10 seconds Rest		Rest for 10 seconds.
	(3) 20 seconds High Knees	Legs, Cardio, Core	Run in place lifting knees high. Repeat for 20 seconds.
	(4) 10 seconds Rest		Rest for 10 seconds.
	4 Rounds for time:		
	(1) 15 Kettlebell Clean	Shoulders, Back, Core	Lift kettlebell to shoulder, flip grip at top. Repeat for 15 reps.
139	(2) 20 V-Ups	Abs, Core, Hip Flexors	Lie back, lift legs and torso simultaneously. Repeat for 20 reps.
	(3) 20 Kettlebell Goblet Squats	Legs, Glutes, Core	Squat holding kettlebell close to chest. Repeat for 20 reps.
	(4) 250-meter run	Legs, Cardio, Core	Run 250 meters at a steady pace.
	Repeat 4 times with 1-minute rest between rounds:		
	(1) 30 seconds Kettlebell Swing	Lower Body, Core, Shoulders	Swing kettlebell between legs, thrust hips forward, raise kettlebell to shoulder height. Repeat for 30 seconds.
140	(2) 30 seconds Push-Ups	Chest, Triceps, Core	Lower body to ground, push up with arms. Repeat for 30 seconds.
	(3) 30 seconds Kettlebell Goblet Squats	Legs, Glutes, Core	Squat holding kettlebell close to chest. Repeat for 30 seconds.
	(4) 30 seconds Mountain Climbers	Cardio, Core, Legs	Run in place in plank position, drive knees to chest. Repeat for 30 seconds.

Workout No.	Workout (Kettlebell & Body-Weight Workouts)	Main Muscle Groups	Instructions
	4 Rounds for time:		
	(1) 15 Kettlebell Swings	Lower Body, Core, Shoulders	Swing kettlebell between legs, thrust hips forward. Repeat for 15 reps.
141	(2) 20 Air Squats	Legs, Glutes, Core	Stand, bend knees to lower body. Repeat for 20 reps.
	(3) 12 Kettlebell Clean and Press	Shoulders, Arms, Core	Clean kettlebell to shoulder, press overhead. Repeat for 12 reps each arm.
	(4) 400-meter run	Legs, Cardio, Core	Run 400 meters at a steady pace.
	Repeat 4 times with 1-minute rest between rounds:		
	(1) 30 seconds Kettlebell Snatch	Shoulders, Back, Core	Lift kettlebell overhead in one motion. Alternate arms. Repeat for 30 seconds.
142	(2) 30 seconds Mountain Climbers	Cardio, Core, Legs	Run in place in plank position, drive knees to chest. Repeat for 30 seconds.
	(3) 30 seconds Kettlebell Thrusters	Shoulders, Legs, Core	Squat to overhead press in one fluid motion. Repeat for 30 seconds.
	(4) 30 seconds Jumping Jacks	Cardio, Legs, Core	Jump to spread legs and clap hands overhead. Repeat for 30 seconds.
	3 Rounds for time:		
	(1) 12 Kettlebell Deadlifts	Lower Back, Hamstrings, Glutes	Lift kettlebell from ground, keep back straight. Repeat for 12 reps.
143	(2) 20 Push-Ups	Chest, Triceps, Core	Lower body to ground, push up with arms. Repeat for 20 reps.
	(3) 15 Kettlebell Bent Over Rows	Back, Shoulders, Arms	Hinge forward, row kettlebell to hip. Repeat for 15 reps each side.
	(4) 500-meter run	Legs, Cardio, Core	Run 500 meters at a steady pace.
	Repeat 5 times:		
	(1) 40 seconds Kettlebell Around the Body	Core, Shoulders, Arms	Pass kettlebell around body, maintain core control. Repeat for 40 seconds.
144	(2) 20 seconds Rest		Rest for 20 seconds.
	(3) 40 seconds Burpees	Full Body, Core, Legs	Jump, squat down, kick back into push-up, return up. Repeat for 40 seconds.
	(4) 20 seconds Rest		Rest for 20 seconds.
	4 Rounds for time:		
	(1) 20 Kettlebell Snatches	Shoulders, Back, Core	Lift kettlebell overhead in one motion. Alternate arms. Repeat for 20 reps each arm.
145	(2) 20 Lunges	Legs, Glutes, Core	Step forward, lower hips to drop knee to ground. Repeat for 20 reps.
	(3) 20 Kettlebell Goblet Squats	Legs, Glutes, Core	Squat holding kettlebell close to chest. Repeat for 20 reps.
	(4) 300-meter run	Legs, Cardio, Core	Run 300 meters at a steady pace.

Workout No.	Workout (Kettlebell & Body-Weight Workouts)		Main Muscle Groups	Instructions
	Repeat 5 times:			
		45 seconds Kettlebell Jump Swing	Legs, Core, Shoulders	Explosive swing with a jump at top of motion. Repeat for 45 seconds.
146		15 seconds Rest		Rest for 15 seconds.
		45 seconds Jumping Jacks	Cardio, Legs, Core	Jump to spread legs and clap hands overhead. Repeat for 45 seconds.
		15 seconds Rest		Rest for 15 seconds.
	3 Rounds for time:			
	(1)	10 Kettlebell Clean and Press	Shoulders, Arms, Core	Clean kettlebell to shoulder, press overhead. Repeat for 10 reps each arm.
147	(2)	20 Push-Ups	Chest, Triceps, Core	Lower body to ground, push up with arms. Repeat for 20 reps.
	(3)	15 Kettlebell Deadlifts	Lower Back, Hamstrings, Glutes	Lift kettlebell from ground, keep back straight. Repeat for 15 reps.
	(4)	300-meter run	Legs, Cardio, Core	Run 300 meters at a steady pace.
	Repeat 8 times:			
	(1)	20 seconds Kettlebell Atlas Swing	Shoulders, Back, Core	Swing kettlebell up, catch at chest level. Repeat for 20 seconds.
148	(2)	10 seconds Rest		Rest for 10 seconds.
	(3)	20 seconds High Knees	Legs, Cardio, Core	Run in place lifting knees high. Repeat for 20 seconds.
	(4)	10 seconds Rest		Rest for 10 seconds.
	4 Rounds for time:			
	(1)	15 Kettlebell Clean	Shoulders, Back, Core	Lift kettlebell to shoulder, flip grip at top. Repeat for 15 reps.
149	(2)	20 V-Ups	Abs, Core, Hip Flexors	Lie back, lift legs and torso simultaneously. Repeat for 20 reps.
	(3)	20 Kettlebell Goblet Squats	Legs, Glutes, Core	Squat holding kettlebell close to chest. Repeat for 20 reps.
	(4)	250-meter run	Legs, Cardio, Core	Run 250 meters at a steady pace.
	Repeat 4 times with 1-minute rest between rounds:			
	(1)	30 seconds Kettlebell Swing	Lower Body, Core, Shoulders	Swing kettlebell between legs, thrust hips forward, raise kettlebell to shoulder height. Repeat for 30 seconds.
150	(2)	30 seconds Push-Ups	Chest, Triceps, Core	Lower body to ground, push up with arms. Repeat for 30 seconds.
	(3)	30 seconds Kettlebell Goblet Squats	Legs, Glutes, Core	Squat holding kettlebell close to chest. Repeat for 30 seconds.
	(4)	30 seconds Mountain Climbers	Cardio, Core, Legs	Run in place in plank position, drive knees to chest. Repeat for 30 seconds.

Workout No.	Workout (Kettlebell ONLY workouts)	Main Muscle Groups	Instructions
1	**As many rounds as possible in 10 mins of:**		
	(1) 10 Goblet Squats	Quads, Glutes, Core	Hold kettlebell at chest, squat, keep back straight.
	(2) 10 Kettlebell Swings	Hamstrings, Glutes, Shoulders	Swing kettlebell to chest height, hinge at hips.
	(3) 10 Push Press	Shoulders, Triceps, Core	Push kettlebell overhead, lock out arms.
2	**Every minute on the minute for 20 mins:**		
	(1) 15 Kettlebell Snatches (Alternating)	Shoulders, Glutes, Hamstrings	Lift kettlebell overhead in one motion, switch hands.
	(2) 20 Russian Twists	Obliques, Core, Shoulders	Twist torso, touch kettlebell to ground each side.
3	**3 Rounds for time:**		
	(1) 15 Kettlebell Cleans	Shoulders, Biceps, Core	Lift kettlebell to shoulder, flip grip at top.
	(2) 20 Kettlebell Deadlifts	Hamstrings, Glutes, Back	Lift kettlebell from ground, keep back straight.
	(3) 15 Pushups on Kettlebell	Chest, Triceps, Shoulders	Perform pushup with hands on kettlebell.
4	**45 secs work / 15 secs rest per exercise for 4 rounds:**		
	(1) Kettlebell Thrusters	Quads, Shoulders, Triceps	Squat to overhead press, one fluid motion.
	(2) Bent Over Rows	Back, Biceps, Core	Row kettlebell to hip, switch sides.
	(3) Kettlebell Jump Swings	Hamstrings, Glutes, Core	Swing kettlebell with a jump at top of motion.
5	**5 Rounds for time:**		
	(1) 10 Turkish GetUps	Shoulders, Core, Legs	Stand from floor, kettlebell overhead, controlled motion.
	(2) 15 Goblet Squats	Quads, Glutes, Core	Hold kettlebell at chest, squat, keep back straight.
	(3) 10 Burpees over Kettlebell	Full Body, Cardio	Perform burpee, jump over kettlebell.

Workout No.	Workout (Kettlebell ONLY workouts)	Main Muscle Groups	Instructions
	As many rounds as possible in 10 mins:		
6	(1) 20 Kettlebell Swings	Hamstrings, Glutes, Shoulders	Swing kettlebell to chest height, hinge at hips.
	(2) 15 Kettlebell Lunges (Alternating)	Quads, Glutes, Core	Step forward into lunge, hold kettlebell for balance.
	(3) 10 Renegade Rows	Back, Biceps, Core	Row kettlebells alternately in plank position.
	21-15-9 Reps for time:		
7	(1) Kettlebell Cleans	Shoulders, Biceps, Core	Lift kettlebell to shoulder, flip grip at top.
	(2) Kettlebell Swings	Hamstrings, Glutes, Shoulders	Swing kettlebell to chest height, hinge at hips.
	(3) Kettlebell Push Press	Shoulders, Triceps, Core	Push kettlebell overhead, lock out arms.
	Every minute on the minute for 25 mins:		
8	(1) 20 Kettlebell Deadlifts	Hamstrings, Glutes, Back	Lift kettlebell from ground, keep back straight.
	(2) 20 Alternating Kettlebell Lunges	Quads, Glutes, Core	Step forward into lunge, hold kettlebell for balance.
	(3) 10 Kettlebell Thrusters	Quads, Shoulders, Triceps	Squat to overhead press, one fluid motion.
	As many rounds as possible in 12 mins:		
9	(1) 10 Goblet Squats	Quads, Glutes, Core	Hold kettlebell at chest, squat, keep back straight.
	(2) 15 Russian Twists	Obliques, Core, Shoulders	Twist torso, touch kettlebell to ground each side.
	(3) 10 Kettlebell Snatches	Shoulders, Glutes, Hamstrings	Lift kettlebell overhead in one motion, switch hands.
	4 Rounds for time:		
10	(1) 10 Kettlebell Thrusters	Quads, Shoulders, Triceps	Squat to overhead press, one fluid motion.
	(2) 15 Bent Over Rows	Back, Biceps, Core	Row kettlebell to hip, switch sides.
	(3) 20 Russian Twists	Obliques, Core, Shoulders	Twist torso, touch kettlebell to ground each side.

Workout No.	Workout (Kettlebell ONLY workouts)	Main Muscle Groups	Instructions
	As many rounds as possible in 12 min:		
11	(1) 10 Goblet Squats	Quads, Glutes, Core	Hold kettlebell at chest, squat, keep back straight.
	(2) 10 Kettlebell Swings	Hamstrings, Glutes, Shoulders	Swing kettlebell to chest height, hinge at hips.
	(3) 10 Push Press	Shoulders, Triceps, Core	Push kettlebell overhead, lock out arms.
	Every minute on the minute for 20 mins:		
12	(1) 15 Kettlebell Snatches (Alternating)	Shoulders, Glutes, Hamstrings	Lift kettlebell overhead in one motion, switch hands.
	(2) 20 Russian Twists	Obliques, Core, Shoulders	Twist torso, touch kettlebell to ground each side.
	3 Rounds for time:		
13	(1) 15 Kettlebell Cleans	Shoulders, Biceps, Core	Lift kettlebell to shoulder, flip grip at top.
	(2) 20 Kettlebell Deadlifts	Hamstrings, Glutes, Back	Lift kettlebell from ground, keep back straight.
	(3) 15 Pushups on Kettlebell	Chest, Triceps, Shoulders	Perform pushup with hands on kettlebell.
	45 secs work / 15 secs rest per exercise for 4 rounds:		
14	(1) Kettlebell Thrusters	Quads, Shoulders, Triceps	Squat to overhead press, one fluid motion.
	(2) Bent Over Rows	Back, Biceps, Core	Row kettlebell to hip, switch sides.
	(3) Kettlebell Jump Swings	Hamstrings, Glutes, Core	Swing kettlebell with a jump at top of motion.
	5 Rounds for time:		
15	(1) 10 Turkish GetUps	Shoulders, Core, Legs	Stand from floor, kettlebell overhead, controlled motion.
	(2) 15 Goblet Squats	Quads, Glutes, Core	Hold kettlebell at chest, squat, keep back straight
	(3) 10 Burpees over Kettlebell	Full Body, Cardio	Perform burpee, jump over kettlebell.

Workout No.	Workout (Kettlebell ONLY workouts)		Main Muscle Groups	Instructions
16	**As many rounds as possible in 10 mins:**			
	(1)	20 Kettlebell Swings	Hamstrings, Glutes, Shoulders	Swing kettlebell to chest height, hinge at hips.
	(2)	15 Kettlebell Lunges (Alternating)	Quads, Glutes, Core	Step forward into lunge, hold kettlebell for balance.
	(3)	10 Renegade Rows	Back, Biceps, Core	Row kettlebells alternately in plank position.
17	**21-15-9 Reps for time:**			
	(1)	Kettlebell Cleans	Shoulders, Biceps, Core	Lift kettlebell to shoulder, flip grip at top.
	(2)	Kettlebell Swings	Hamstrings, Glutes, Shoulders	Swing kettlebell to chest height, hinge at hips.
	(3)	Kettlebell Push Press	Shoulders, Triceps, Core	Push kettlebell overhead, lock out arms.
18	**Every minute on the minute for 25 mins:**			
	(1)	20 Kettlebell Deadlifts	Hamstrings, Glutes, Back	Lift kettlebell from ground, keep back straight.
	(2)	20 Alternating Kettlebell Lunges	Quads, Glutes, Core	Step forward into lunge, hold kettlebell for balance.
	(3)	10 Kettlebell Thrusters	Quads, Shoulders, Triceps	Squat to overhead press, one fluid motion.
19	**As many rounds as possible in 12 mins:**			
	(1)	10 Goblet Squats	Quads, Glutes, Core	Hold kettlebell at chest, squat, keep back straight.
	(2)	15 Russian Twists	Obliques, Core, Shoulders	Twist torso, touch kettlebell to ground each side.
	(3)	10 Kettlebell Snatches	Shoulders, Glutes, Hamstrings	Lift kettlebell overhead in one motion, switch hands.
20	**4 Rounds for time:**			
	(1)	10 Kettlebell Thrusters	Quads, Shoulders, Triceps	Squat to overhead press, one fluid motion.
	(2)	15 Bent Over Rows	Back, Biceps, Core	Row kettlebell to hip, switch sides.
	(3)	20 Russian Twists	Obliques, Core, Shoulders	Twist torso, touch kettlebell to ground each side.

Workout No.	Workout (Kettlebell ONLY workouts)	Main Muscle Groups	Instructions
	As many rounds as possible in 15 min:		
21	(1) 10 Goblet Squats	Quads, Glutes, Core	Hold kettlebell at chest, squat, keep back straight.
	(2) 10 Kettlebell Swings	Hamstrings, Glutes, Shoulders	Swing kettlebell to chest height, hinge at hips.
	(3) 10 Push Press	Shoulders, Triceps, Core	Push kettlebell overhead, lock out arms.
	Every minute on the minute for 20 mins:		
22	(1) 12 Kettlebell Snatches (Alternating)	Shoulders, Glutes, Hamstrings	Lift kettlebell overhead in one motion, switch hands.
	(2) 16 Russian Twists	Obliques, Core, Shoulders	Twist torso, touch kettlebell to ground each side.
	4 Rounds for time:		
23	(1) 20 Kettlebell Cleans	Shoulders, Biceps, Core	Lift kettlebell to shoulder, flip grip at top.
	(2) 15 Kettlebell Deadlifts	Hamstrings, Glutes, Back	Lift kettlebell from ground, keep back straight.
	(3) 20 Pushups on Kettlebell	Chest, Triceps, Shoulders	Perform pushup with hands on kettlebell.
	45 secs work / 15 secs rest per exercise for 5 rounds:		
24	(1) Kettlebell Thrusters	Quads, Shoulders, Triceps	Squat to overhead press, one fluid motion.
	(2) Bent Over Rows	Back, Biceps, Core	Row kettlebell to hip, switch sides.
	(3) Kettlebell Jump Swings	Hamstrings, Glutes, Core	Swing kettlebell with a jump at top of motion.
	5 Rounds for time:		
25	(1) 10 Turkish GetUps	Shoulders, Core, Legs	Stand from floor, kettlebell overhead, controlled motion.
	(2) 20 Goblet Squats	Quads, Glutes, Core	Hold kettlebell at chest, squat, keep back straight.
	(3) 15 Burpees over Kettlebell	Full Body, Cardio	Perform burpee, jump over kettlebell.

Workout No.	Workout (Kettlebell ONLY workouts)	Main Muscle Groups	Instructions
	As many rounds as possible in 12 mins:		
26	(1) 15 Kettlebell Swings	Hamstrings, Glutes, Shoulders	Swing kettlebell to chest height, hinge at hips.
	(2) 12 Kettlebell Lunges (Alternating)	Quads, Glutes, Core	Step forward into lunge, hold kettlebell for balance.
	(3) 10 Renegade Rows	Back, Biceps, Core	Row kettlebells alternately in plank position.
	21-15-9 Reps for time:		
27	(1) Kettlebell Cleans	Shoulders, Biceps, Core	Lift kettlebell to shoulder, flip grip at top.
	(2) Kettlebell Swings	Hamstrings, Glutes, Shoulders	Swing kettlebell to chest height, hinge at hips.
	(3) Kettlebell Push Press	Shoulders, Triceps, Core	Push kettlebell overhead, lock out arms.
	Every minute on the minute for 25 mins:		
28	(1) 15 Kettlebell Deadlifts	Hamstrings, Glutes, Back	Lift kettlebell from ground, keep back straight.
	(2) 12 Alternating Kettlebell Lunges	Quads, Glutes, Core	Step forward into lunge, hold kettlebell for balance.
	(3) 10 Kettlebell Thrusters	Quads, Shoulders, Triceps	Squat to overhead press, one fluid motion.
	As many rounds as possible in 12 mins:		
29	(1) 10 Goblet Squats	Quads, Glutes, Core	Hold kettlebell at chest, squat, keep back straight.
	(2) 20 Russian Twists	Obliques, Core, Shoulders	Twist torso, touch kettlebell to ground each side.
	(3) 15 Kettlebell Snatches	Shoulders, Glutes, Hamstrings	Lift kettlebell overhead in one motion, switch hands.
	5 Rounds for time:		
30	(1) 12 Kettlebell Thrusters	Quads, Shoulders, Triceps	Squat to overhead press, one fluid motion.
	(2) 15 Bent Over Rows	Back, Biceps, Core	Row kettlebell to hip, switch sides.
	(3) 20 Russian Twists	Obliques, Core, Shoulders	Twist torso, touch kettlebell to ground each side.

Workout No.	Workout (Kettlebell ONLY workouts)	Main Muscle Groups	Instructions
	As many rounds as possible in 12 min:		
31	(1) 12 Goblet Squats	Quads, Glutes, Core	Hold kettlebell at chest, squat, keep back straight.
	(2) 15 Kettlebell Swings	Hamstrings, Glutes, Shoulders	Swing kettlebell to chest height, hinge at hips.
	(3) 10 Push Press	Shoulders, Triceps, Core	Push kettlebell overhead, lock out arms.
	Every minute on the minute for 20 mins:		
32	(1) 12 Kettlebell Snatches (Alternating)	Shoulders, Glutes, Hamstrings	Lift kettlebell overhead in one motion, switch hands.
	(2) 16 Russian Twists	Obliques, Core, Shoulders	Twist torso, touch kettlebell to ground each side.
	3 Rounds for time:		
33	(1) 15 Kettlebell Cleans	Shoulders, Biceps, Core	Lift kettlebell to shoulder, flip grip at top.
	(2) 20 Kettlebell Deadlifts	Hamstrings, Glutes, Back	Lift kettlebell from ground, keep back straight.
	(3) 15 Pushups on Kettlebell	Chest, Triceps, Shoulders	Perform pushup with hands on kettlebell.
	45 secs work / 15 secs rest per exercise for 4 rounds:		
34	(1) Kettlebell Thrusters	Quads, Shoulders, Triceps	Squat to overhead press, one fluid motion.
	(2) Bent Over Rows	Back, Biceps, Core	Row kettlebell to hip, switch sides.
	(3) Kettlebell Jump Swings	Hamstrings, Glutes, Core	Swing kettlebell with a jump at top of motion.
	5 Rounds for time:		
35	(1) 10 Turkish GetUps	Shoulders, Core, Legs	Stand from floor, kettlebell overhead, controlled motion.
	(2) 15 Goblet Squats	Quads, Glutes, Core	Hold kettlebell at chest, squat, keep back straight.
	(3) 10 Burpees over Kettlebell	Full Body, Cardio	Perform burpee, jump over kettlebell.

Workout No.	Workout (Kettlebell ONLY workouts)		Main Muscle Groups	Instructions
	As many rounds as possible in 10 mins:			
36	(1)	20 Kettlebell Swings	Hamstrings, Glutes, Shoulders	Swing kettlebell to chest height, hinge at hips.
	(2)	15 Kettlebell Lunges (Alternating)	Quads, Glutes, Core	Step forward into lunge, hold kettlebell for balance.
	(3)	10 Renegade Rows	Back, Biceps, Core	Row kettlebells alternately in plank position.
	21-15-9 Reps for time:			
37	(1)	Kettlebell Cleans	Shoulders, Biceps, Core	Lift kettlebell to shoulder, flip grip at top.
	(2)	Kettlebell Swings	Hamstrings, Glutes, Shoulders	Swing kettlebell to chest height, hinge at hips.
	(3)	Kettlebell Push Press	Shoulders, Triceps, Core	Push kettlebell overhead, lock out arms.
	Every minute on the minute for 25 mins:			
38	(1)	20 Kettlebell Deadlifts	Hamstrings, Glutes, Back	Lift kettlebell from ground, keep back straight.
	(2)	20 Alternating Kettlebell Lunges	Quads, Glutes, Core	Step forward into lunge, hold kettlebell for balance.
	(3)	10 Kettlebell Thrusters	Quads, Shoulders, Triceps	Squat to overhead press, one fluid motion.
	As many rounds as possible in 12 mins:			
39	(1)	10 Goblet Squats	Quads, Glutes, Core	Hold kettlebell at chest, squat, keep back straight.
	(2)	15 Russian Twists	Obliques, Core, Shoulders	Twist torso, touch kettlebell to ground each side.
	(3)	10 Kettlebell Snatches	Shoulders, Glutes, Hamstrings	Lift kettlebell overhead in one motion, switch hands.
	4 Rounds for time:			
40	(1)	10 Kettlebell Thrusters	Quads, Shoulders, Triceps	Squat to overhead press, one fluid motion.
	(2)	15 Bent Over Rows	Back, Biceps, Core	Row kettlebell to hip, switch sides.
	(3)	20 Russian Twists	Obliques, Core, Shoulders	Twist torso, touch kettlebell to ground each side.

Workout No.	Workout (Kettlebell ONLY workouts)	Main Muscle Groups	Instructions
	As many rounds as possible in 12 min:		
41	(1) 15 Goblet Squats	Quads, Glutes, Core	Hold kettlebell at chest, squat, keep back straight.
	(2) 12 Kettlebell Swings	Hamstrings, Glutes, Shoulders	Swing kettlebell to chest height, hinge at hips.
	(3) 10 Push Press	Shoulders, Triceps, Core	Push kettlebell overhead, lock out arms.
	Every minute on the minute for 20 mins:		
42	(1) 12 Kettlebell Snatches (Alternating)	Shoulders, Glutes, Hamstrings	Lift kettlebell overhead in one motion, switch hands.
	(2) 16 Russian Twists	Obliques, Core, Shoulders	Twist torso, touch kettlebell to ground each side.
	3 Rounds for time:		
43	(1) 15 Kettlebell Cleans	Shoulders, Biceps, Core	Lift kettlebell to shoulder, flip grip at top.
	(2) 20 Kettlebell Deadlifts	Hamstrings, Glutes, Back	Lift kettlebell from ground, keep back straight.
	(3) 15 Pushups on Kettlebell	Chest, Triceps, Shoulders	Perform pushup with hands on kettlebell.
	45 secs work / 15 secs rest per exercise for 4 rounds:		
44	(1) Kettlebell Thrusters	Quads, Shoulders, Triceps	Squat to overhead press, one fluid motion.
	(2) Bent Over Rows	Back, Biceps, Core	Row kettlebell to hip, switch sides.
	(3) Kettlebell Jump Swings	Hamstrings, Glutes, Core	Swing kettlebell with a jump at top of motion.
	5 Rounds for time:		
45	(1) 10 Turkish GetUps	Shoulders, Core, Legs	Stand from floor, kettlebell overhead, controlled motion.
	(2) 15 Goblet Squats	Quads, Glutes, Core	Hold kettlebell at chest, squat, keep back straight.
	(3) 10 Burpees over Kettlebell	Full Body, Cardio	Perform burpee, jump over kettlebell.

Workout No.	Workout (Kettlebell ONLY workouts)		Main Muscle Groups	Instructions
	As many rounds as possible in 10 mins:			
46	(1)	20 Kettlebell Swings	Hamstrings, Glutes, Shoulders	Swing kettlebell to chest height, hinge at hips.
	(2)	15 Kettlebell Lunges (Alternating)	Quads, Glutes, Core	Step forward into lunge, hold kettlebell for balance.
	(3)	10 Renegade Rows	Back, Biceps, Core	Row kettlebells alternately in plank position.
	21-15-9 Reps for time:			
47	(1)	Kettlebell Cleans	Shoulders, Biceps, Core	Lift kettlebell to shoulder, flip grip at top.
	(2)	Kettlebell Swings	Hamstrings, Glutes, Shoulders	Swing kettlebell to chest height, hinge at hips.
	(3)	Kettlebell Push Press	Shoulders, Triceps, Core	Push kettlebell overhead, lock out arms.
	Every minute on the minute for 25 mins:			
48	(1)	20 Kettlebell Deadlifts	Hamstrings, Glutes, Back	Lift kettlebell from ground, keep back straight.
	(2)	20 Alternating Kettlebell Lunges	Quads, Glutes, Core	Step forward into lunge, hold kettlebell for balance.
	(3)	10 Kettlebell Thrusters	Quads, Shoulders, Triceps	Squat to overhead press, one fluid motion.
	As many rounds as possible in 12 mins:			
49	(1)	10 Goblet Squats	Quads, Glutes, Core	Hold kettlebell at chest, squat, keep back straight.
	(2)	15 Russian Twists	Obliques, Core, Shoulders	Twist torso, touch kettlebell to ground each side.
	(3)	10 Kettlebell Snatches	Shoulders, Glutes, Hamstrings	Lift kettlebell overhead in one motion, switch hands.
	4 Rounds for time:			
50	(1)	10 Kettlebell Thrusters	Quads, Shoulders, Triceps	Squat to overhead press, one fluid motion.
	(2)	15 Bent Over Rows	Back, Biceps, Core	Row kettlebell to hip, switch sides.
	(3)	20 Russian Twists	Obliques, Core, Shoulders	Twist torso, touch kettlebell to ground each side.

Workout No.	Workout (Kettlebell ONLY workouts)		Main Muscle Groups	Instructions
	As many rounds as possible in 15 min:			
51	(1)	15 Goblet Squats	Quads, Glutes, Core	Hold kettlebell at chest, squat, keep back straight.
	(2)	12 Kettlebell Swings	Hamstrings, Glutes, Shoulders	Swing kettlebell to chest height, hinge at hips.
	(3)	10 Push Press	Shoulders, Triceps, Core	Push kettlebell overhead, lock out arms.
	Every minute on the minute for 20 mins:			
52	(1)	12 Kettlebell Snatches (Alternating)	Shoulders, Glutes, Hamstrings	Lift kettlebell overhead in one motion, switch hands.
	(2)	16 Russian Twists	Obliques, Core, Shoulders	Twist torso, touch kettlebell to ground each side.
	3 Rounds for time:			
53	(1)	15 Kettlebell Cleans	Shoulders, Biceps, Core	Lift kettlebell to shoulder, flip grip at top.
	(2)	20 Kettlebell Deadlifts	Hamstrings, Glutes, Back	Lift kettlebell from ground, keep back straight.
	(3)	15 Pushups on Kettlebell	Chest, Triceps, Shoulders	Perform pushup with hands on kettlebell.
	45 secs work / 15 secs rest per exercise for 4 rounds:			
54	(1)	Kettlebell Thrusters	Quads, Shoulders, Triceps	Squat to overhead press, one fluid motion.
	(2)	Bent Over Rows	Back, Biceps, Core	Row kettlebell to hip, switch sides.
	(3)	Kettlebell Jump Swings	Hamstrings, Glutes, Core	Swing kettlebell with a jump at top of motion.
	5 Rounds for time:			
55	(1)	10 Turkish GetUps	Shoulders, Core, Legs	Stand from floor, kettlebell overhead, controlled motion.
	(2)	15 Goblet Squats	Quads, Glutes, Core	Hold kettlebell at chest, squat, keep back straight.
	(3)	10 Burpees over Kettlebell	Full Body, Cardio	Perform burpee, jump over kettlebell.

Workout No.	Workout (Kettlebell ONLY workouts)	Main Muscle Groups	Instructions
	As many rounds as possible in 10 mins:		
56	(1) 20 Kettlebell Swings	Hamstrings, Glutes, Shoulders	Swing kettlebell to chest height, hinge at hips.
	(2) 15 Kettlebell Lunges (Alternating)	Quads, Glutes, Core	Step forward into lunge, hold kettlebell for balance.
	(3) 10 Renegade Rows	Back, Biceps, Core	Row kettlebells alternately in plank position.
	21-15-9 Reps for time:		
57	(1) Kettlebell Cleans	Shoulders, Biceps, Core	Lift kettlebell to shoulder, flip grip at top.
	(2) Kettlebell Swings	Hamstrings, Glutes, Shoulders	Swing kettlebell to chest height, hinge at hips.
	(3) Kettlebell Push Press	Shoulders, Triceps, Core	Push kettlebell overhead, lock out arms.
	Every minute on the minute for 25 mins:		
58	(1) 20 Kettlebell Deadlifts	Hamstrings, Glutes, Back	Lift kettlebell from ground, keep back straight.
	(2) 20 Alternating Kettlebell Lunges	Quads, Glutes, Core	Step forward into lunge, hold kettlebell for balance.
	(3) 10 Kettlebell Thrusters	Quads, Shoulders, Triceps	Squat to overhead press, one fluid motion.
	As many rounds as possible in 12 mins:		
59	(1) 10 Goblet Squats	Quads, Glutes, Core	Hold kettlebell at chest, squat, keep back straight.
	(2) 15 Russian Twists	Obliques, Core, Shoulders	Twist torso, touch kettlebell to ground each side.
	(3) 10 Kettlebell Snatches	Shoulders, Glutes, Hamstrings	Lift kettlebell overhead in one motion, switch hands.
	4 Rounds for time:		
60	(1) 10 Kettlebell Thrusters	Quads, Shoulders, Triceps	Squat to overhead press, one fluid motion.
	(2) 15 Bent Over Rows	Back, Biceps, Core	Row kettlebell to hip, switch sides.
	(3) 20 Russian Twists	Obliques, Core, Shoulders	Twist torso, touch kettlebell to ground each side.

Workout No.	Workout (Kettlebell ONLY workouts)		Main Muscle Groups	Instructions
61		**As many rounds as possible in 15 min:**		
	(1)	15 Goblet Squats	Quads, Glutes, Core	Hold kettlebell at chest, squat, keep back straight.
	(2)	12 Kettlebell Swings	Hamstrings, Glutes, Shoulders	Swing kettlebell to chest height, hinge at hips.
	(3)	10 Push Press	Shoulders, Triceps, Core	Push kettlebell overhead, lock out arms.
62		**Every minute on the minute for 20 mins:**		
	(1)	12 Kettlebell Snatches (Alternating)	Shoulders, Glutes, Hamstrings	Lift kettlebell overhead in one motion, switch hands.
	(2)	16 Russian Twists	Obliques, Core, Shoulders	Twist torso, touch kettlebell to ground each side.
63		**3 Rounds for time:**		
	(1)	15 Kettlebell Cleans	Shoulders, Biceps, Core	Lift kettlebell to shoulder, flip grip at top.
	(2)	20 Kettlebell Deadlifts	Hamstrings, Glutes, Back	Lift kettlebell from ground, keep back straight.
	(3)	15 Pushups on Kettlebell	Chest, Triceps, Shoulders	Perform pushup with hands on kettlebell.
64		**45 secs work / 15 secs rest per exercise for 4 rounds:**		
	(1)	Kettlebell Thrusters	Quads, Shoulders, Triceps	Squat to overhead press, one fluid motion.
	(2)	Bent Over Rows	Back, Biceps, Core	Row kettlebell to hip, switch sides.
	(3)	Kettlebell Jump Swings	Hamstrings, Glutes, Core	Swing kettlebell with a jump at top of motion.
65		**5 Rounds for time:**		
	(1)	10 Turkish GetUps	Shoulders, Core, Legs	Stand from floor, kettlebell overhead, controlled motion.
	(2)	15 Goblet Squats	Quads, Glutes, Core	Hold kettlebell at chest, squat, keep back straight.
	(3)	10 Burpees over Kettlebell	Full Body, Cardio	Perform burpee, jump over kettlebell.

Workout No.	Workout (Kettlebell ONLY workouts)		Main Muscle Groups	Instructions
66	**As many rounds as possible in 10 mins:**			
	(1)	20 Kettlebell Swings	Hamstrings, Glutes, Shoulders	Swing kettlebell to chest height, hinge at hips.
	(2)	15 Kettlebell Lunges (Alternating)	Quads, Glutes, Core	Step forward into lunge, hold kettlebell for balance.
	(3)	10 Renegade Rows	Back, Biceps, Core	Row kettlebells alternately in plank position.
67	**21-15-9 Reps for time:**			
	(1)	Kettlebell Cleans	Shoulders, Biceps, Core	Lift kettlebell to shoulder, flip grip at top.
	(2)	Kettlebell Swings	Hamstrings, Glutes, Shoulders	Swing kettlebell to chest height, hinge at hips.
	(3)	Kettlebell Push Press	Shoulders, Triceps, Core	Push kettlebell overhead, lock out arms.
68	**Every minute on the minute for 25 mins:**			
	(1)	20 Kettlebell Deadlifts	Hamstrings, Glutes, Back	Lift kettlebell from ground, keep back straight.
	(2)	20 Alternating Kettlebell Lunges	Quads, Glutes, Core	Step forward into lunge, hold kettlebell for balance.
	(3)	10 Kettlebell Thrusters	Quads, Shoulders, Triceps	Squat to overhead press, one fluid motion.
69	**As many rounds as possible in 12 mins:**			
	(1)	10 Goblet Squats	Quads, Glutes, Core	Hold kettlebell at chest, squat, keep back straight.
	(2)	15 Russian Twists	Obliques, Core, Shoulders	Twist torso, touch kettlebell to ground each side.
	(3)	10 Kettlebell Snatches	Shoulders, Glutes, Hamstrings	Lift kettlebell overhead in one motion, switch hands.
70	**4 Rounds for time:**			
	(1)	10 Kettlebell Thrusters	Quads, Shoulders, Triceps	Squat to overhead press, one fluid motion.
	(2)	15 Bent Over Rows	Back, Biceps, Core	Row kettlebell to hip, switch sides.
	(3)	20 Russian Twists	Obliques, Core, Shoulders	Twist torso, touch kettlebell to ground each side.

Workout No.	Workout (Kettlebell ONLY workouts)	Main Muscle Groups	Instructions
	As many rounds as possible in 15 min:		
71	(1) 15 Goblet Squats	Quads, Glutes, Core	Hold kettlebell at chest, squat, keep back straight.
	(2) 12 Kettlebell Swings	Hamstrings, Glutes, Shoulders	Swing kettlebell to chest height, hinge at hips.
	(3) 10 Push Press	Shoulders, Triceps, Core	Push kettlebell overhead, lock out arms.
	Every minute on the minute for 20 mins:		
72	(1) 12 Kettlebell Snatches (Alternating)	Shoulders, Glutes, Hamstrings	Lift kettlebell overhead in one motion, switch hands.
	(2) 16 Russian Twists	Obliques, Core, Shoulders	Twist torso, touch kettlebell to ground each side.
	3 Rounds for time:		
73	(1) 15 Kettlebell Cleans	Shoulders, Biceps, Core	Lift kettlebell to shoulder, flip grip at top.
	(2) 20 Kettlebell Deadlifts	Hamstrings, Glutes, Back	Lift kettlebell from ground, keep back straight.
	(3) 15 Pushups on Kettlebell	Chest, Triceps, Shoulders	Perform pushup with hands on kettlebell.
	45 secs work / 15 secs rest per exercise for 4 rounds:		
74	(1) Kettlebell Thrusters	Quads, Shoulders, Triceps	Squat to overhead press, one fluid motion.
	(2) Bent Over Rows	Back, Biceps, Core	Row kettlebell to hip, switch sides.
	(3) Kettlebell Jump Swings	Hamstrings, Glutes, Core	Swing kettlebell with a jump at top of motion.
	5 Rounds for time:		
75	(1) 10 Turkish GetUps	Shoulders, Core, Legs	Stand from floor, kettlebell overhead, controlled motion.
	(2) 15 Goblet Squats	Quads, Glutes, Core	Hold kettlebell at chest, squat, keep back straight.
	(3) 10 Burpees over Kettlebell	Full Body, Cardio	Perform burpee, jump over kettlebell.

Workout No.	Workout (Kettlebell ONLY workouts)	Main Muscle Groups	Instructions
	As many rounds as possible in 10 mins:		
76	(1) 20 Kettlebell Swings	Hamstrings, Glutes, Shoulders	Swing kettlebell to chest height, hinge at hips.
	(2) 15 Kettlebell Lunges (Alternating)	Quads, Glutes, Core	Step forward into lunge, hold kettlebell for balance.
	(3) 10 Renegade Rows	Back, Biceps, Core	Row kettlebells alternately in plank position.
	21-15-9 Reps for time:		
77	(1) Kettlebell Cleans	Shoulders, Biceps, Core	Lift kettlebell to shoulder, flip grip at top.
	(2) Kettlebell Swings	Hamstrings, Glutes, Shoulders	Swing kettlebell to chest height, hinge at hips.
	(3) Kettlebell Push Press	Shoulders, Triceps, Core	Push kettlebell overhead, lock out arms.
	Every minute on the minute for 25 mins:		
78	(1) 20 Kettlebell Deadlifts	Hamstrings, Glutes, Back	Lift kettlebell from ground, keep back straight.
	(2) 20 Alternating Kettlebell Lunges	Quads, Glutes, Core	Step forward into lunge, hold kettlebell for balance.
	(3) 10 Kettlebell Thrusters	Quads, Shoulders, Triceps	Squat to overhead press, one fluid motion.
	As many rounds as possible in 12 mins:		
79	(1) 10 Goblet Squats	Quads, Glutes, Core	Hold kettlebell at chest, squat, keep back straight.
	(2) 15 Russian Twists	Obliques, Core, Shoulders	Twist torso, touch kettlebell to ground each side.
	(3) 10 Kettlebell Snatches	Shoulders, Glutes, Hamstrings	Lift kettlebell overhead in one motion, switch hands.
	4 Rounds for time:		
80	(1) 10 Kettlebell Thrusters	Quads, Shoulders, Triceps	Squat to overhead press, one fluid motion.
	(2) 15 Bent Over Rows	Back, Biceps, Core	Row kettlebell to hip, switch sides.
	(3) 20 Russian Twists	Obliques, Core, Shoulders	Twist torso, touch kettlebell to ground each side.

Workout No.	Workout (Kettlebell ONLY workouts)	Main Muscle Groups	Instructions
	As many rounds as possible in 15 min:		
81	(1) 15 Goblet Squats	Quads, Glutes, Core	Hold kettlebell at chest, squat, keep back straight.
	(2) 12 Kettlebell Swings	Hamstrings, Glutes, Shoulders	Swing kettlebell to chest height, hinge at hips.
	(3) 10 Push Press	Shoulders, Triceps, Core	Push kettlebell overhead, lock out arms.
	Every minute on the minute for 20 mins:		
82	(1) 12 Kettlebell Snatches (Alternating)	Shoulders, Glutes, Hamstrings	Lift kettlebell overhead in one motion, switch hands.
	(2) 16 Russian Twists	Obliques, Core, Shoulders	Twist torso, touch kettlebell to ground each side.
	3 Rounds for time:		
83	(1) 15 Kettlebell Cleans	Shoulders, Biceps, Core	Lift kettlebell to shoulder, flip grip at top.
	(2) 20 Kettlebell Deadlifts	Hamstrings, Glutes, Back	Lift kettlebell from ground, keep back straight.
	(3) 15 Pushups on Kettlebell	Chest, Triceps, Shoulders	Perform pushup with hands on kettlebell.
	45 secs work / 15 secs rest per exercise for 4 rounds:		
84	(1) Kettlebell Thrusters	Quads, Shoulders, Triceps	Squat to overhead press, one fluid motion.
	(2) Bent Over Rows	Back, Biceps, Core	Row kettlebell to hip, switch sides.
	(3) Kettlebell Jump Swings	Hamstrings, Glutes, Core	Swing kettlebell with a jump at top of motion.
	5 Rounds for time:		
85	(1) 10 Turkish GetUps	Shoulders, Core, Legs	Stand from floor, kettlebell overhead, controlled motion.
	(2) 15 Goblet Squats	Quads, Glutes, Core	Hold kettlebell at chest, squat, keep back straight.
	(3) 10 Burpees over Kettlebell	Full Body, Cardio	Perform burpee, jump over kettlebell.

Workout No.	Workout (Kettlebell ONLY workouts)	Main Muscle Groups	Instructions
	As many rounds as possible in 10 mins:		
86	(1) 20 Kettlebell Swings	Hamstrings, Glutes, Shoulders	Swing kettlebell to chest height, hinge at hips.
	(2) 15 Kettlebell Lunges (Alternating)	Quads, Glutes, Core	Step forward into lunge, hold kettlebell for balance.
	(3) 10 Renegade Rows	Back, Biceps, Core	Row kettlebells alternately in plank position.
	21-15-9 Reps for time:		
87	(1) Kettlebell Cleans	Shoulders, Biceps, Core	Lift kettlebell to shoulder, flip grip at top.
	(2) Kettlebell Swings	Hamstrings, Glutes, Shoulders	Swing kettlebell to chest height, hinge at hips.
	(3) Kettlebell Push Press	Shoulders, Triceps, Core	Push kettlebell overhead, lock out arms.
	Every minute on the minute for 25 mins:		
88	(1) 20 Kettlebell Deadlifts	Hamstrings, Glutes, Back	Lift kettlebell from ground, keep back straight.
	(2) 20 Alternating Kettlebell Lunges	Quads, Glutes, Core	Step forward into lunge, hold kettlebell for balance.
	(3) 10 Kettlebell Thrusters	Quads, Shoulders, Triceps	Squat to overhead press, one fluid motion.
	As many rounds as possible in 12 mins:		
89	(1) 10 Goblet Squats	Quads, Glutes, Core	Hold kettlebell at chest, squat, keep back straight.
	(2) 15 Russian Twists	Obliques, Core, Shoulders	Twist torso, touch kettlebell to ground each side.
	(3) 10 Kettlebell Snatches	Shoulders, Glutes, Hamstrings	Lift kettlebell overhead in one motion, switch hands.
	4 Rounds for time:		
90	(1) 10 Kettlebell Thrusters	Quads, Shoulders, Triceps	Squat to overhead press, one fluid motion.
	(2) 15 Bent Over Rows	Back, Biceps, Core	Row kettlebell to hip, switch sides.
	(3) 20 Russian Twists	Obliques, Core, Shoulders	Twist torso, touch kettlebell to ground each side.

Workout No.	Workout (Kettlebell ONLY workouts)	Main Muscle Groups	Instructions
	As many rounds as possible in 15 min:		
91	(1) 15 Goblet Squats	Quads, Glutes, Core	Hold kettlebell at chest, squat, keep back straight.
	(2) 12 Kettlebell Swings	Hamstrings, Glutes, Shoulders	Swing kettlebell to chest height, hinge at hips.
	(3) 10 Push Press	Shoulders, Triceps, Core	Push kettlebell overhead, lock out arms.
	Every minute on the minute for 20 mins:		
92	(1) 12 Kettlebell Snatches (Alternating)	Shoulders, Glutes, Hamstrings	Lift kettlebell overhead in one motion, switch hands.
	(2) 16 Russian Twists	Obliques, Core, Shoulders	Twist torso, touch kettlebell to ground each side.
	3 Rounds for time:		
93	(1) 15 Kettlebell Cleans	Shoulders, Biceps, Core	Lift kettlebell to shoulder, flip grip at top.
	(2) 20 Kettlebell Deadlifts	Hamstrings, Glutes, Back	Lift kettlebell from ground, keep back straight.
	(3) 15 Pushups on Kettlebell	Chest, Triceps, Shoulders	Perform pushup with hands on kettlebell.
	45 secs work / 15 secs rest per exercise for 4 rounds:		
94	(1) Kettlebell Thrusters	Quads, Shoulders, Triceps	Squat to overhead press, one fluid motion.
	(2) Bent Over Rows	Back, Biceps, Core	Row kettlebell to hip, switch sides.
	(3) Kettlebell Jump Swings	Hamstrings, Glutes, Core	Swing kettlebell with a jump at top of motion.
	5 Rounds for time:		
95	(1) 10 Turkish GetUps	Shoulders, Core, Legs	Stand from floor, kettlebell overhead, controlled motion.
	(2) 15 Goblet Squats	Quads, Glutes, Core	Hold kettlebell at chest, squat, keep back straight.
	(3) 10 Burpees over Kettlebell	Full Body, Cardio	Perform burpee, jump over kettlebell.

Workout No.	Workout (Kettlebell ONLY workouts)	Main Muscle Groups	Instructions
	As many rounds as possible in 10 mins:		
96	(1) 20 Kettlebell Swings	Hamstrings, Glutes, Shoulders	Swing kettlebell to chest height, hinge at hips.
	(2) 15 Kettlebell Lunges (Alternating)	Quads, Glutes, Core	Step forward into lunge, hold kettlebell for balance.
	(3) 10 Renegade Rows	Back, Biceps, Core	Row kettlebells alternately in plank position.
	21-15-9 Reps for time:		
97	(1) Kettlebell Cleans	Shoulders, Biceps, Core	Lift kettlebell to shoulder, flip grip at top.
	(2) Kettlebell Swings	Hamstrings, Glutes, Shoulders	Swing kettlebell to chest height, hinge at hips.
	(3) Kettlebell Push Press	Shoulders, Triceps, Core	Push kettlebell overhead, lock out arms.
	Every minute on the minute for 25 mins:		
98	(1) 20 Kettlebell Deadlifts	Hamstrings, Glutes, Back	Lift kettlebell from ground, keep back straight.
	(2) 20 Alternating Kettlebell Lunges	Quads, Glutes, Core	Step forward into lunge, hold kettlebell for balance.
	(3) 10 Kettlebell Thrusters	Quads, Shoulders, Triceps	Squat to overhead press, one fluid motion.
	As many rounds as possible in 12 mins:		
99	(1) 10 Goblet Squats	Quads, Glutes, Core	Hold kettlebell at chest, squat, keep back straight.
	(2) 15 Russian Twists	Obliques, Core, Shoulders	Twist torso, touch kettlebell to ground each side.
	(3) 10 Kettlebell Snatches	Shoulders, Glutes, Hamstrings	Lift kettlebell overhead in one motion, switch hands.
	4 Rounds for time:		
100	(1) 10 Kettlebell Thrusters	Quads, Shoulders, Triceps	Squat to overhead press, one fluid motion.
	(2) 15 Bent Over Rows	Back, Biceps, Core	Row kettlebell to hip, switch sides.
	(3) 20 Russian Twists	Obliques, Core, Shoulders	Twist torso, touch kettlebell to ground each side.

Workout No.	Workout (Kettlebell ONLY workouts)	Main Muscle Groups	Instructions
	As many rounds as possible in 15 min:		
101	(1) 15 Goblet Squats	Quads, Glutes, Core	Hold kettlebell at chest, squat, keep back straight.
	(2) 12 Kettlebell Swings	Hamstrings, Glutes, Shoulders	Swing kettlebell to chest height, hinge at hips.
	(3) 10 Push Press	Shoulders, Triceps, Core	Push kettlebell overhead, lock out arms.
	Every minute on the minute for 20 mins:		
102	(1) 12 Kettlebell Snatches (Alternating)	Shoulders, Glutes, Hamstrings	Lift kettlebell overhead in one motion, switch hands.
	(2) 16 Russian Twists	Obliques, Core, Shoulders	Twist torso, touch kettlebell to ground each side.
	3 Rounds for time:		
103	(1) 15 Kettlebell Cleans	Shoulders, Biceps, Core	Lift kettlebell to shoulder, flip grip at top.
	(2) 20 Kettlebell Deadlifts	Hamstrings, Glutes, Back	Lift kettlebell from ground, keep back straight.
	(3) 15 Pushups on Kettlebell	Chest, Triceps, Shoulders	Perform pushup with hands on kettlebell.
	45 secs work / 15 secs rest per exercise for 4 rounds:		
104	(1) Kettlebell Thrusters	Quads, Shoulders, Triceps	Squat to overhead press, one fluid motion.
	(2) Bent Over Rows	Back, Biceps, Core	Row kettlebell to hip, switch sides.
	(3) Kettlebell Jump Swings	Hamstrings, Glutes, Core	Swing kettlebell with a jump at top of motion.
	5 Rounds for time:		
105	(1) 10 Turkish GetUps	Shoulders, Core, Legs	Stand from floor, kettlebell overhead, controlled motion.
	(2) 15 Goblet Squats	Quads, Glutes, Core	Hold kettlebell at chest, squat, keep back straight.
	(3) 10 Burpees over Kettlebell	Full Body, Cardio	Perform burpee, jump over kettlebell.

Workout No.	Workout (Kettlebell ONLY workouts)	Main Muscle Groups	Instructions
	As many rounds as possible in 10 mins:		
106	(1) 20 Kettlebell Swings	Hamstrings, Glutes, Shoulders	Swing kettlebell to chest height, hinge at hips.
	(2) 15 Kettlebell Lunges (Alternating)	Quads, Glutes, Core	Step forward into lunge, hold kettlebell for balance.
	(3) 10 Renegade Rows	Back, Biceps, Core	Row kettlebells alternately in plank position.
	21-15-9 Reps for time:		
107	(1) Kettlebell Cleans	Shoulders, Biceps, Core	Lift kettlebell to shoulder, flip grip at top.
	(2) Kettlebell Swings	Hamstrings, Glutes, Shoulders	Swing kettlebell to chest height, hinge at hips.
	(3) Kettlebell Push Press	Shoulders, Triceps, Core	Push kettlebell overhead, lock out arms.
	Every minute on the minute for 25 mins:		
108	(1) 20 Kettlebell Deadlifts	Hamstrings, Glutes, Back	Lift kettlebell from ground, keep back straight.
	(2) 20 Alternating Kettlebell Lunges	Quads, Glutes, Core	Step forward into lunge, hold kettlebell for balance.
	(3) 10 Kettlebell Thrusters	Quads, Shoulders, Triceps	Squat to overhead press, one fluid motion.
	As many rounds as possible in 12 mins:		
109	(1) 10 Goblet Squats	Quads, Glutes, Core	Hold kettlebell at chest, squat, keep back straight.
	(2) 15 Russian Twists	Obliques, Core, Shoulders	Twist torso, touch kettlebell to ground each side.
	(3) 10 Kettlebell Snatches	Shoulders, Glutes, Hamstrings	Lift kettlebell overhead in one motion, switch hands.
	4 Rounds for time:		
110	(1) 10 Kettlebell Thrusters	Quads, Shoulders, Triceps	Squat to overhead press, one fluid motion.
	(2) 15 Bent Over Rows	Back, Biceps, Core	Row kettlebell to hip, switch sides.
	(3) 20 Russian Twists	Obliques, Core, Shoulders	Twist torso, touch kettlebell to ground each side.

Workout No.	Workout (Kettlebell ONLY workouts)	Main Muscle Groups	Instructions
	As many rounds as possible in 15 min:		
111	(1) 15 Goblet Squats	Quads, Glutes, Core	Hold kettlebell at chest, squat, keep back straight.
	(2) 12 Kettlebell Swings	Hamstrings, Glutes, Shoulders	Swing kettlebell to chest height, hinge at hips.
	(3) 10 Push Press	Shoulders, Triceps, Core	Push kettlebell overhead, lock out arms.
	Every minute on the minute for 20 mins:		
112	(1) 12 Kettlebell Snatches (Alternating)	Shoulders, Glutes, Hamstrings	Lift kettlebell overhead in one motion, switch hands.
	(2) 16 Russian Twists	Obliques, Core, Shoulders	Twist torso, touch kettlebell to ground each side.
	3 Rounds for time:		
113	(1) 15 Kettlebell Cleans	Shoulders, Biceps, Core	Lift kettlebell to shoulder, flip grip at top.
	(2) 20 Kettlebell Deadlifts	Hamstrings, Glutes, Back	Lift kettlebell from ground, keep back straight.
	(3) 15 Pushups on Kettlebell	Chest, Triceps, Shoulders	Perform pushup with hands on kettlebell.
	45 secs work / 15 secs rest per exercise for 4 rounds:		
114	(1) Kettlebell Thrusters	Quads, Shoulders, Triceps	Squat to overhead press, one fluid motion.
	(2) Bent Over Rows	Back, Biceps, Core	Row kettlebell to hip, switch sides.
	(3) Kettlebell Jump Swings	Hamstrings, Glutes, Core	Swing kettlebell with a jump at top of motion.
	5 Rounds for time:		
115	(1) 10 Turkish GetUps	Shoulders, Core, Legs	Stand from floor, kettlebell overhead, controlled motion.
	(2) 15 Goblet Squats	Quads, Glutes, Core	Hold kettlebell at chest, squat, keep back straight.
	(3) 10 Burpees over Kettlebell	Full Body, Cardio	Perform burpee, jump over kettlebell.

Workout No.	Workout (Kettlebell ONLY workouts)	Main Muscle Groups	Instructions
	As many rounds as possible in 10 mins:		
116	(1) 20 Kettlebell Swings	Hamstrings, Glutes, Shoulders	Swing kettlebell to chest height, hinge at hips.
	(2) 15 Kettlebell Lunges (Alternating)	Quads, Glutes, Core	Step forward into lunge, hold kettlebell for balance.
	(3) 10 Renegade Rows	Back, Biceps, Core	Row kettlebells alternately in plank position.
	21-15-9 Reps for time:		
117	(1) Kettlebell Cleans	Shoulders, Biceps, Core	Lift kettlebell to shoulder, flip grip at top.
	(2) Kettlebell Swings	Hamstrings, Glutes, Shoulders	Swing kettlebell to chest height, hinge at hips.
	(3) Kettlebell Push Press	Shoulders, Triceps, Core	Push kettlebell overhead, lock out arms.
	Every minute on the minute for 25 mins:		
118	(1) 20 Kettlebell Deadlifts	Hamstrings, Glutes, Back	Lift kettlebell from ground, keep back straight.
	(2) 20 Alternating Kettlebell Lunges	Quads, Glutes, Core	Step forward into lunge, hold kettlebell for balance.
	(3) 10 Kettlebell Thrusters	Quads, Shoulders, Triceps	Squat to overhead press, one fluid motion.
	As many rounds as possible in 12 mins:		
119	(1) 10 Goblet Squats	Quads, Glutes, Core	Hold kettlebell at chest, squat, keep back straight.
	(2) 15 Russian Twists	Obliques, Core, Shoulders	Twist torso, touch kettlebell to ground each side.
	(3) 10 Kettlebell Snatches	Shoulders, Glutes, Hamstrings	Lift kettlebell overhead in one motion, switch hands.
	4 Rounds for time:		
120	(1) 10 Kettlebell Thrusters	Quads, Shoulders, Triceps	Squat to overhead press, one fluid motion.
	(2) 15 Bent Over Rows	Back, Biceps, Core	Row kettlebell to hip, switch sides.
	(3) 20 Russian Twists	Obliques, Core, Shoulders	Twist torso, touch kettlebell to ground each side.

Workout No.	Workout (Kettlebell ONLY workouts)	Main Muscle Groups	Instructions
	As many rounds as possible in 12 min:		
121	(1) 15 Goblet Squats	Quads, Glutes, Core	Hold kettlebell at chest, squat, keep back straight.
	(2) 10 Kettlebell Swings	Hamstrings, Glutes, Shoulders	Swing kettlebell to chest height, hinge at hips.
	(3) 5 Push Press	Shoulders, Triceps, Core	Push kettlebell overhead, lock out arms.
	Every minute on the minute for 20 mins:		
122	(1) 12 Kettlebell Snatches (Alternating)	Shoulders, Glutes, Hamstrings	Lift kettlebell overhead in one motion, switch hands.
	(2) 15 Russian Twists	Obliques, Core, Shoulders	Twist torso, touch kettlebell to ground each side.
	5 Rounds for time:		
123	(1) 15 Kettlebell Cleans	Shoulders, Biceps, Core	Lift kettlebell to shoulder, flip grip at top.
	(2) 20 Kettlebell Deadlifts	Hamstrings, Glutes, Back	Lift kettlebell from ground, keep back straight.
	(3) 15 Pushups on Kettlebell	Chest, Triceps, Shoulders	Perform pushup with hands on kettlebell.
	45 secs work / 15 secs rest per exercise for 4 rounds:		
124	(1) Kettlebell Thrusters	Quads, Shoulders, Triceps	Squat to overhead press, one fluid motion.
	(2) Bent Over Rows	Back, Biceps, Core	Row kettlebell to hip, switch sides.
	(3) Kettlebell Jump Swings	Hamstrings, Glutes, Core	Swing kettlebell with a jump at top of motion.
	4 Rounds for time:		
125	(1) 10 Turkish GetUps	Shoulders, Core, Legs	Stand from floor, kettlebell overhead, controlled motion.
	(2) 15 Goblet Squats	Quads, Glutes, Core	Hold kettlebell at chest, squat, keep back straight.
	(3) 10 Burpees over Kettlebell	Full Body, Cardio	Perform burpee, jump over kettlebell.

Workout No.	Workout (Kettlebell ONLY workouts)		Main Muscle Groups	Instructions
	As many rounds as possible in 10 mins:			
126	(1)	20 Kettlebell Swings	Hamstrings, Glutes, Shoulders	Swing kettlebell to chest height, hinge at hips.
	(2)	15 Kettlebell Lunges (Alternating)	Quads, Glutes, Core	Step forward into lunge, hold kettlebell for balance.
	(3)	10 Renegade Rows	Back, Biceps, Core	Row kettlebells alternately in plank position.
	21-15-9 Reps for time:			
127	(1)	Kettlebell Cleans	Shoulders, Biceps, Core	Lift kettlebell to shoulder, flip grip at top.
	(2)	Kettlebell Swings	Hamstrings, Glutes, Shoulders	Swing kettlebell to chest height, hinge at hips.
	(3)	Kettlebell Push Press	Shoulders, Triceps, Core	Push kettlebell overhead, lock out arms.
	Every minute on the minute for 25 mins:			
128	(1)	20 Kettlebell Deadlifts	Hamstrings, Glutes, Back	Lift kettlebell from ground, keep back straight.
	(2)	20 Alternating Kettlebell Lunges	Quads, Glutes, Core	Step forward into lunge, hold kettlebell for balance.
	(3)	10 Kettlebell Thrusters	Quads, Shoulders, Triceps	Squat to overhead press, one fluid motion.
	As many rounds as possible in 12 mins:			
129	(1)	10 Goblet Squats	Quads, Glutes, Core	Hold kettlebell at chest, squat, keep back straight.
	(2)	15 Russian Twists	Obliques, Core, Shoulders	Twist torso, touch kettlebell to ground each side.
	(3)	10 Kettlebell Snatches	Shoulders, Glutes, Hamstrings	Lift kettlebell overhead in one motion, switch hands.
	4 Rounds for time:			
130	(1)	10 Kettlebell Thrusters	Quads, Shoulders, Triceps	Squat to overhead press, one fluid motion.
	(2)	15 Bent Over Rows	Back, Biceps, Core	Row kettlebell to hip, switch sides.
	(3)	20 Russian Twists	Obliques, Core, Shoulders	Twist torso, touch kettlebell to ground each side.

Workout No.	Workout (Kettlebell ONLY workouts)	Main Muscle Groups	Instructions
131	**As many rounds as possible in 10 min:**		
	(1) 15 Goblet Squats	Quads, Glutes, Core	Hold kettlebell at chest, squat, keep back straight.
	(2) 10 Kettlebell Swings	Hamstrings, Glutes, Shoulders	Swing kettlebell to chest height, hinge at hips.
	(3) 5 Push Press	Shoulders, Triceps, Core	Push kettlebell overhead, lock out arms.
132	**Every minute on the minute for 20 mins:**		
	(1) 12 Kettlebell Snatches (Alternating)	Shoulders, Glutes, Hamstrings	Lift kettlebell overhead in one motion, switch hands.
	(2) 15 Russian Twists	Obliques, Core, Shoulders	Twist torso, touch kettlebell to ground each side.
133	**5 Rounds for time:**		
	(1) 15 Kettlebell Cleans	Shoulders, Biceps, Core	Lift kettlebell to shoulder, flip grip at top.
	(2) 20 Kettlebell Deadlifts	Hamstrings, Glutes, Back	Lift kettlebell from ground, keep back straight.
	(3) 15 Pushups on Kettlebell	Chest, Triceps, Shoulders	Perform pushup with hands on kettlebell.
134	**45 secs work / 15 secs rest per exercise for 4 rounds:**		
	(1) Kettlebell Thrusters	Quads, Shoulders, Triceps	Squat to overhead press, one fluid motion.
	(2) Bent Over Rows	Back, Biceps, Core	Row kettlebell to hip, switch sides.
	(3) Kettlebell Jump Swings	Hamstrings, Glutes, Core	Swing kettlebell with a jump at top of motion.
135	**4 Rounds for time:**		
	(1) 10 Turkish GetUps	Shoulders, Core, Legs	Stand from floor, kettlebell overhead, controlled motion.
	(2) 15 Goblet Squats	Quads, Glutes, Core	Hold kettlebell at chest, squat, keep back straight.
	(3) 10 Burpees over Kettlebell	Full Body, Cardio	Perform burpee, jump over kettlebell.

Workout No.	Workout (Kettlebell ONLY workouts)	Main Muscle Groups	Instructions
	As many rounds as possible in 10 mins:		
136	(1) 20 Kettlebell Swings	Hamstrings, Glutes, Shoulders	Swing kettlebell to chest height, hinge at hips.
	(2) 15 Kettlebell Lunges (Alternating)	Quads, Glutes, Core	Step forward into lunge, hold kettlebell for balance.
	(3) 10 Renegade Rows	Back, Biceps, Core	Row kettlebells alternately in plank position.
	21-15-9 Reps for time:		
137	(1) Kettlebell Cleans	Shoulders, Biceps, Core	Lift kettlebell to shoulder, flip grip at top.
	(2) Kettlebell Swings	Hamstrings, Glutes, Shoulders	Swing kettlebell to chest height, hinge at hips.
	(3) Kettlebell Push Press	Shoulders, Triceps, Core	Push kettlebell overhead, lock out arms.
	Every minute on the minute for 25 mins:		
138	(1) 20 Kettlebell Deadlifts	Hamstrings, Glutes, Back	Lift kettlebell from ground, keep back straight.
	(2) 20 Alternating Kettlebell Lunges	Quads, Glutes, Core	Step forward into lunge, hold kettlebell for balance.
	(3) 10 Kettlebell Thrusters	Quads, Shoulders, Triceps	Squat to overhead press, one fluid motion.
	As many rounds as possible in 12 mins:		
139	(1) 10 Goblet Squats	Quads, Glutes, Core	Hold kettlebell at chest, squat, keep back straight.
	(2) 15 Russian Twists	Obliques, Core, Shoulders	Twist torso, touch kettlebell to ground each side.
	(3) 10 Kettlebell Snatches	Shoulders, Glutes, Hamstrings	Lift kettlebell overhead in one motion, switch hands.
	4 Rounds for time:		
140	(1) 10 Kettlebell Thrusters	Quads, Shoulders, Triceps	Squat to overhead press, one fluid motion.
	(2) 15 Bent Over Rows	Back, Biceps, Core	Row kettlebell to hip, switch sides.
	(3) 20 Russian Twists	Obliques, Core, Shoulders	Twist torso, touch kettlebell to ground each side.

Workout No.	Workout (Kettlebell ONLY workouts)	Main Muscle Groups	Instructions
	As many rounds as possible in 15 min:		
141	(1) 15 Goblet Squats	Quads, Glutes, Core	Hold kettlebell at chest, squat, keep back straight.
	(2) 10 Kettlebell Swings	Hamstrings, Glutes, Shoulders	Swing kettlebell to chest height, hinge at hips.
	(3) 5 Push Press	Shoulders, Triceps, Core	Push kettlebell overhead, lock out arms.
	Every minute on the minute for 20 mins:		
142	(1) 12 Kettlebell Snatches (Alternating)	Shoulders, Glutes, Hamstrings	Lift kettlebell overhead in one motion, switch hands.
	(2) 15 Russian Twists	Obliques, Core, Shoulders	Twist torso, touch kettlebell to ground each side.
	5 Rounds for time:		
143	(1) 15 Kettlebell Cleans	Shoulders, Biceps, Core	Lift kettlebell to shoulder, flip grip at top.
	(2) 20 Kettlebell Deadlifts	Hamstrings, Glutes, Back	Lift kettlebell from ground, keep back straight.
	(3) 15 Pushups on Kettlebell	Chest, Triceps, Shoulders	Perform pushup with hands on kettlebell.
	45 secs work / 15 secs rest per exercise for 4 rounds:		
144	(1) Kettlebell Thrusters	Quads, Shoulders, Triceps	Squat to overhead press, one fluid motion.
	(2) Bent Over Rows	Back, Biceps, Core	Row kettlebell to hip, switch sides.
	(3) Kettlebell Jump Swings	Hamstrings, Glutes, Core	Swing kettlebell with a jump at top of motion.
	4 Rounds for time:		
145	(1) 10 Turkish GetUps	Shoulders, Core, Legs	Stand from floor, kettlebell overhead, controlled motion.
	(2) 15 Goblet Squats	Quads, Glutes, Core	Hold kettlebell at chest, squat, keep back straight.
	(3) 10 Burpees over Kettlebell	Full Body, Cardio	Perform burpee, jump over kettlebell.

Workout No.	Workout (Kettlebell ONLY workouts)	Main Muscle Groups	Instructions
	As many rounds as possible in 10 mins:		
146	(1) 20 Kettlebell Swings	Hamstrings, Glutes, Shoulders	Swing kettlebell to chest height, hinge at hips.
	(2) 15 Kettlebell Lunges (Alternating)	Quads, Glutes, Core	Step forward into lunge, hold kettlebell for balance.
	(3) 10 Renegade Rows	Back, Biceps, Core	Row kettlebells alternately in plank position.
	21-15-9 Reps for time:		
147	(1) Kettlebell Cleans	Shoulders, Biceps, Core	Lift kettlebell to shoulder, flip grip at top.
	(2) Kettlebell Swings	Hamstrings, Glutes, Shoulders	Swing kettlebell to chest height, hinge at hips.
	(3) Kettlebell Push Press	Shoulders, Triceps, Core	Push kettlebell overhead, lock out arms.
	Every minute on the minute for 25 mins:		
148	(1) 20 Kettlebell Deadlifts	Hamstrings, Glutes, Back	Lift kettlebell from ground, keep back straight.
	(2) 20 Alternating Kettlebell Lunges	Quads, Glutes, Core	Step forward into lunge, hold kettlebell for balance.
	(3) 10 Kettlebell Thrusters	Quads, Shoulders, Triceps	Squat to overhead press, one fluid motion.
	As many rounds as possible in 12 mins:		
149	(1) 10 Goblet Squats	Quads, Glutes, Core	Hold kettlebell at chest, squat, keep back straight.
	(2) 15 Russian Twists	Obliques, Core, Shoulders	Twist torso, touch kettlebell to ground each side.
	(3) 10 Kettlebell Snatches	Shoulders, Glutes, Hamstrings	Lift kettlebell overhead in one motion, switch hands.
	4 Rounds for time:		
150	(1) 10 Kettlebell Thrusters	Quads, Shoulders, Triceps	Squat to overhead press, one fluid motion.
	(2) 15 Bent Over Rows	Back, Biceps, Core	Row kettlebell to hip, switch sides.
	(3) 20 Russian Twists	Obliques, Core, Shoulders	Twist torso, touch kettlebell to ground each side.

Kettlebell Exercises

ALTERNATING CURL

Curl kettlebells alternately, focus on bicep isolation.

1. Stand with feet shoulder-width apart, holding a kettlebell in each hand.
2. Keep your elbows close to your torso and your palms facing forward.
3. Curl the right kettlebell while keeping the left arm stationary.
4. Lower the right kettlebell back to the starting position.
5. Repeat the movement with the left kettlebell.
6. Continue alternating curls, focusing on bicep isolation.

AROUND THE BODY

Pass kettlebell around body, maintain core control.

1. Stand with feet hip-width apart, holding a kettlebell in front of you.
2. Pass the kettlebell around your body, starting from the front.
3. Keep your core engaged to maintain balance.
4. Transfer the kettlebell from one hand to the other behind your back.
5. Continue the motion, passing the kettlebell around your body in a circular motion.
6. Reverse the direction halfway through the set.

ATLAS SWING

Swing kettlebell up, catch at chest level.

1. Stand with feet shoulder-width apart, holding a kettlebell in one hand.
2. Swing the kettlebell between your legs.
3. Drive your hips forward to swing the kettlebell up to chest level.
4. Catch the kettlebell with your other hand at chest height.
5. Swing the kettlebell back down and repeat the motion.
6. Switch hands after completing the set.

BENT OVER ROW

Hinge forward, row kettlebell to hip, switch sides.

1. Stand with feet hip-width apart, holding a kettlebell in each hand.
2. Hinge forward at the hips, keeping your back straight.
3. Let the kettlebells hang directly under your shoulders.
4. Row the right kettlebell to your hip, squeezing your shoulder blade.
5. Lower the right kettlebell and repeat with the left kettlebell.
6. Alternate sides, maintaining a controlled movement.

BOB AND WEAVE

Duck and weave sideways
holding kettlebell.

1. Stand with feet shoulder-width apart, holding a kettlebell with both hands.
2. Bend your knees slightly and engage your core.
3. Duck down to the right, keeping the kettlebell close to your chest.
4. Weave under an imaginary obstacle, moving to the left.
5. Stand up on the left side and repeat the movement to the right.
6. Continue ducking and weaving, maintaining a smooth rhythm.

CHEST PRESS

Press kettlebell from chest
while lying down.

1. Lie on your back with your knees bent and feet flat on the floor.
2. Hold a kettlebell in each hand, with your elbows bent and close to your body.
3. Press the kettlebells straight up, extending your arms fully.
4. Lower the kettlebells back down to your chest.
5. Keep your movements controlled and your core engaged.
6. Repeat the press, focusing on chest muscle engagement.

CLEAN

Lift kettlebell to shoulder,
flip grip at top.

1. Stand with feet shoulder-width apart, holding a kettlebell in one hand.
2. Bend your knees and lower the kettlebell between your legs.
3. Drive through your heels and extend your hips to pull the kettlebell up.
4. Flip your grip at the top, catching the kettlebell on the back of your wrist.
5. Lower the kettlebell back down to the starting position.
6. Repeat the movement, focusing on a smooth, controlled lift.

CURL

Curl kettlebell using standard grip,
focus on biceps.

1. Stand with feet shoulder-width apart, holding a kettlebell in each hand.
2. Keep your elbows close to your torso and your palms facing inward.
3. Curl both kettlebells simultaneously, focusing on your biceps.
4. Lower the kettlebells back to the starting position.
5. Maintain a controlled movement throughout the exercise.
6. Repeat the curls, ensuring full range of motion.

DEADLIFT

Lift kettlebell from ground, keep back straight.

1. Stand with feet hip-width apart, kettlebell on the floor between your feet.
2. Hinge at your hips and bend your knees to grasp the kettlebell handle.
3. Keep your back straight, engage your core, and drive through your heels to lift the kettlebell.
4. Stand up fully, keeping the kettlebell close to your body.
5. Reverse the movement to lower the kettlebell back to the ground.
6. Repeat, ensuring proper form throughout.

DECK SQUAT

Squat, roll back, stand up while holding kettlebell.

1. Stand with feet shoulder-width apart, holding a kettlebell close to your chest.
2. Squat down and roll back onto your back, tucking your knees towards your chest.
3. Use momentum to roll forward and stand back up, maintaining the kettlebell at your chest.
4. Keep your core engaged to assist with the movement.
5. Repeat the squat and roll sequence.
6. Focus on smooth transitions between the rolling and standing phases.

DEFICIT PUSH UP

Push-up holding kettlebell to increase depth.

1. Place two kettlebells on the floor shoulder-width apart.
2. Assume a push-up position with hands gripping the kettlebell handles.
3. Lower your body until your chest is in line with the kettlebells.
4. Push through your palms to return to the starting position.
5. Keep your body in a straight line from head to heels.
6. Repeat, maintaining a controlled pace and proper form.

DOUBLE ARM SWING

Swing kettlebell with both hands, hinge at hips.

1. Stand with feet shoulder-width apart, holding a kettlebell with both hands.
2. Hinge at your hips, letting the kettlebell swing back between your legs.
3. Drive your hips forward to swing the kettlebell up to shoulder height.
4. Keep your arms straight but relaxed throughout the movement.
5. Allow the kettlebell to swing back down between your legs.
6. Repeat, maintaining a fluid motion.

FARMER'S WALK

Walk holding kettlebell in each hand, keep back straight.

1. Stand with feet shoulder-width apart, holding a kettlebell in each hand.
2. Engage your core and keep your back straight.
3. Walk forward, maintaining an upright posture.
4. Keep the kettlebells at your sides with your arms straight.
5. Walk for the desired distance or time.
6. Focus on steady, controlled steps.

FIGURE EIGHT

Pass kettlebell through legs in figure-eight motion.

1. Stand with feet wider than shoulder-width apart, holding a kettlebell in one hand.
2. Bend your knees and hinge at your hips to pass the kettlebell between your legs.
3. Grab the kettlebell with the opposite hand behind your leg.
4. Swing the kettlebell around the outside of your leg and pass it through your legs again.
5. Continue the figure-eight motion, alternating hands.
6. Keep your core engaged and maintain a stable stance.

FRONT RAISE

Lift kettlebell to shoulder, flip grip at top.

1. Stand with feet shoulder-width apart, holding a kettlebell in one hand.
2. Keep your arm straight and lift the kettlebell to shoulder height.
3. Flip your grip at the top, rotating the kettlebell.
4. Lower the kettlebell back to the starting position.
5. Repeat the movement, maintaining a controlled pace.
6. Switch hands and repeat for the other side.

GOBLET SQUAT

Squat holding kettlebell close to chest.

1. Stand with feet shoulder-width apart, holding a kettlebell close to your chest with both hands.
2. Engage your core and squat down, keeping your chest up and back straight.
3. Lower your hips until your thighs are parallel to the ground.
4. Drive through your heels to return to the standing position.
5. Keep the kettlebell close to your chest throughout the movement.
6. Repeat, maintaining proper squat form.

GOOD MORNING

Hinge at hips holding kettlebell, focus on hamstrings.

1. Stand with feet shoulder-width apart, holding a kettlebell close to your chest.
2. Hinge at your hips, keeping your back straight and knees slightly bent.
3. Lower your torso until it is parallel to the ground.
4. Engage your hamstrings and glutes to return to the standing position.
5. Keep the kettlebell stable and your core engaged throughout the movement.
6. Repeat, maintaining proper form to avoid strain on your lower back.

HALF TURKISH GET UP

Rise from floor to seated, kettlebell overhead.

1. Lie on your back with your right leg bent and right foot flat on the floor, holding a kettlebell in your right hand.
2. Extend your left arm and leg on the floor.
3. Press the kettlebell straight up, keeping your eyes on it.
4. Roll onto your left forearm, then onto your left hand.
5. Push through your right foot to lift your hips off the ground.
6. Come up to a seated position, maintaining the kettlebell overhead.
7. Reverse the steps to return to the starting position.
8. Repeat on the other side.

HALO

Circle kettlebell around head, maintain posture.

1. Stand with feet shoulder-width apart, holding a kettlebell by the horns at chest level.
2. Circle the kettlebell around your head, starting from the front.
3. Keep your core engaged and your head steady.
4. Complete the circle by bringing the kettlebell back to the starting position.
5. Perform the movement slowly and smoothly to avoid straining your neck.
6. Reverse the direction halfway through the set.

HIP BRIDGE PULLOVER

Hip thrust while pulling kettlebell over chest.

1. Lie on your back with your knees bent and feet flat on the floor, holding a kettlebell with both hands above your chest.
2. Lift your hips into a bridge position, engaging your glutes and core.
3. Slowly lower the kettlebell over your head until your arms are fully extended.
4. Pull the kettlebell back to the starting position above your chest.
5. Lower your hips back to the ground.
6. Repeat, maintaining a controlled movement throughout.

I LEG REV. PLANK

One-leg reverse plank, hold
kettlebell above chest.

1. Sit on the floor with your legs extended and a kettlebell next to you.
2. Place your hands on the ground behind you and lift your hips into a reverse plank position.
3. Raise your right leg off the ground and hold the kettlebell above your chest with both hands.
4. Keep your body in a straight line from head to the left heel.
5. Hold the position for the desired amount of time.
6. Lower your leg and hips, then switch sides.

JUMP SWING

Explosive swing with a
jump at top of motion.

1. Stand with feet shoulder-width apart, holding a kettlebell with both hands.
2. Hinge at your hips, letting the kettlebell swing back between your legs.
3. Drive your hips forward and swing the kettlebell up to shoulder height.
4. At the top of the swing, explosively jump off the ground.
5. Land softly and allow the kettlebell to swing back down between your legs.
6. Repeat the movement, focusing on a smooth transition between the swing and jump.

L SIT & HOLD

Sit, legs straight, hold
kettlebell, maintain L-shape.

1. Sit on the ground with your legs extended straight in front of you.
2. Place a kettlebell on the ground between your legs.
3. Lift your legs and torso off the ground, forming an L shape with your body.
4. Hold the kettlebell with both hands above your chest.
5. Keep your core engaged and maintain the L shape.
6. Hold the position for the desired amount of time.

LEG RAISE

Raise legs while lying down,
hold kettlebell for weight.

1. Lie on your back with your legs extended and a kettlebell held in both hands above your chest.
2. Engage your core and lift your legs off the ground.
3. Raise your legs until they are perpendicular to the floor.
4. Slowly lower your legs back to the starting position without letting them touch the ground.
5. Keep the kettlebell stable and your lower back pressed into the floor.
6. Repeat, maintaining a controlled movement throughout.

LUNGE

Hinge at hips holding kettlebell,
focus on hamstrings.

1. Stand with feet shoulder-width apart,
   holding a kettlebell with both hands.
2. Step forward with your right foot and
   lower your hips, bending both knees to
   90 degrees.
3. Keep your back straight and core
   engaged.
4. Push through your right heel to return
   to the starting position.
5. Repeat on the left leg.
6. Focus on keeping your weight evenly
   distributed and maintaining balance.

LUNGE PASS

Pass kettlebell under leg
during lunge.

1. Stand with feet hip-width apart,
   holding a kettlebell in your right hand.
2. Step forward with your left foot into a
   lunge position.
3. Pass the kettlebell under your left
   thigh to your left hand.
4. Push through your left heel to return to
   the starting position.
5. Repeat on the other side, passing the
   kettlebell under your right thigh.
6. Maintain a controlled motion, ensuring
   a stable core.

LUNGE PRESS

Lunge, press kettlebell
overhead simultaneously.

1. Stand with feet shoulder-width apart,
   holding a kettlebell in your right hand.
2. Step forward with your left foot into a
   lunge position.
3. As you lower into the lunge, press the
   kettlebell overhead.
4. Keep your core engaged and back
   straight.
5. Push through your left heel to return to
   the starting position, lowering the
   kettlebell.
6. Repeat on the other side, ensuring
   synchronized movements.

OVERHEAD SIT UP

Sit-up with kettlebell held
overhead.

1. Lie on your back with legs extended
   and a kettlebell held overhead with
   both hands.
2. Engage your core and sit up, keeping
   the kettlebell overhead.
3. Reach a seated position with your
   torso upright.
4. Slowly lower back down to the starting
   position.
5. Keep your arms extended and the
   kettlebell stable throughout the
   movement.
6. Repeat, focusing on a controlled
   ascent and descent.

OVERHEAD SQUAT

Squat with kettlebell held above head.

1. Stand with feet shoulder-width apart, holding a kettlebell overhead with both hands.
2. Engage your core and squat down, keeping the kettlebell stable.
3. Lower your hips until your thighs are parallel to the ground.
4. Push through your heels to return to the standing position.
5. Keep your back straight and chest up throughout the movement.
6. Repeat, ensuring the kettlebell remains overhead.

PISTOL SQUAT

One-legged squat holding kettlebell for balance.

1. Stand on your right leg, holding a kettlebell in front of your chest with both hands.
2. Extend your left leg forward and lower into a one-legged squat.
3. Keep your chest up and core engaged.
4. Push through your right heel to return to the starting position.
5. Repeat on the left leg.
6. Focus on balance and control throughout the movement.

PLANK PULL THROUGH

Plank, pull kettlebell across floor under chest.

1. Start in a plank position with a kettlebell to the right side of your body.
2. Reach your left hand under your body to pull the kettlebell across to the left side.
3. Return your left hand to the plank position.
4. Repeat with your right hand, pulling the kettlebell back to the right side.
5. Keep your core engaged and hips stable throughout the movement.
6. Continue alternating sides, maintaining a strong plank position.

PULLOVER

Lie back, pull kettlebell from overhead to chest.

1. Lie on your back with knees bent and feet flat on the floor, holding a kettlebell with both hands.
2. Extend your arms overhead, lowering the kettlebell towards the floor.
3. Engage your core and pull the kettlebell back over your chest.
4. Keep your arms slightly bent and the movement controlled.
5. Lower the kettlebell back to the starting position.
6. Repeat, focusing on a smooth, controlled motion.

PUSH-UP

Standard push-up holding
kettlebell handles.

1. Start in a plank position with hands gripping kettlebell handles.
2. Lower your body until your chest touches the ground, keeping elbows close to your body.
3. Engage your core and maintain a straight line from head to heels.
4. Push through your palms to return to the starting position.
5. Repeat, focusing on controlled movements and maintaining proper form.
6. Ensure your shoulders, hips, and feet stay aligned throughout.

RENEGADE

Plank and row kettlebells,
alternating sides.

1. Start in a plank position with a kettlebell in each hand.
2. Row the right kettlebell to your hip while stabilizing your body with your left hand.
3. Lower the right kettlebell back to the ground.
4. Repeat the row with the left kettlebell.
5. Alternate sides, maintaining a strong plank position.
6. Keep your core engaged to prevent hip rotation.

RENEGADE ROW

Row kettlebells alternately
in plank position.

1. Assume a plank position with hands gripping kettlebell handles.
2. Row the right kettlebell to your hip, keeping your body stable.
3. Lower the right kettlebell back to the ground.
4. Repeat the row with the left kettlebell.
5. Alternate sides, maintaining a strong core.
6. Focus on controlled movements and avoid twisting your hips.

RUSSIAN TWIST

Twist torso holding kettlebell,
seated on ground.

1. Sit on the ground with knees bent and feet flat, holding a kettlebell with both hands.
2. Lean back slightly to engage your core and lift your feet off the ground.
3. Twist your torso to the right, bringing the kettlebell beside your hip.
4. Twist to the left, bringing the kettlebell beside your left hip.
5. Continue alternating sides in a controlled motion.
6. Keep your back straight and core engaged throughout.

SHOULDER PRESS

Press kettlebell overhead from shoulder level.

1. Stand with feet shoulder-width apart, holding a kettlebell in one hand at shoulder level.
2. Engage your core and press the kettlebell overhead until your arm is fully extended.
3. Lower the kettlebell back to shoulder level.
4. Repeat the press, maintaining a controlled movement.
5. Switch hands and repeat on the other side.
6. Focus on keeping your body stable and avoiding leaning.

SIDE BEND

Bend sideways holding kettlebell, return upright.

1. Stand with feet shoulder-width apart, holding a kettlebell in your right hand.
2. Place your left hand on your hip and engage your core.
3. Bend sideways to the right, lowering the kettlebell towards your knee.
4. Return to the starting position by engaging your left obliques.
5. Repeat for the desired number of repetitions.
6. Switch sides and repeat the movement.

SIDE LUNGE

Step to side into lunge, kettlebell in hand for weight.

1. Stand with feet together, holding a kettlebell close to your chest.
2. Step to the right into a lunge, bending your right knee and keeping your left leg straight.
3. Push through your right heel to return to the starting position.
4. Repeat on the left side, stepping into a left lunge.
5. Alternate sides, maintaining a strong core and upright posture.
6. Focus on controlled movements and balance.

SIDE PLANK

Hold side plank, lift kettlebell with free hand.

1. Start in a side plank position on your right elbow, with your body forming a straight line.
2. Hold a kettlebell in your left hand, resting it on your hip.
3. Lift the kettlebell towards the ceiling, keeping your arm straight.
4. Lower the kettlebell back to your hip.
5. Maintain the side plank position throughout the movement.
6. Switch sides and repeat the movement on the other side.

SIDE PLANK ROW

Row kettlebell in side plank position, stabilize core.

1. Start in a side plank position on your right elbow, body in a straight line.
2. Hold a kettlebell in your left hand, extended in front of you.
3. Engage your core and row the kettlebell towards your left hip.
4. Keep your body stable, avoiding any hip rotation.
5. Lower the kettlebell back to the starting position.
6. Repeat, then switch sides.

SIDE RAISE

Lift kettlebell laterally to shoulder height.

1. Stand with feet shoulder-width apart, holding a kettlebell in each hand at your sides.
2. Engage your core and raise both kettlebells laterally to shoulder height.
3. Keep a slight bend in your elbows.
4. Lower the kettlebells back to the starting position.
5. Repeat, maintaining a controlled movement.
6. Avoid shrugging your shoulders during the raise.

SIDE SWING

Swing kettlebell side to side, maintain grip.

1. Stand with feet shoulder-width apart, holding a kettlebell in your right hand.
2. Swing the kettlebell to your left side, pivoting on your feet.
3. Allow the kettlebell to swing back to the right side, pivoting your feet in the opposite direction.
4. Keep your core engaged and your movements controlled.
5. Repeat for the desired number of repetitions.
6. Switch hands and repeat the movement.

SIDEWINDER

Move kettlebell in zigzag motion while holding squat.

1. Stand with feet wider than shoulder-width apart, holding a kettlebell with both hands.
2. Lower into a squat position, keeping your back straight.
3. Swing the kettlebell from side to side in a zigzag motion.
4. Maintain the squat position throughout the movement.
5. Keep your core engaged and movements smooth.
6. Repeat for the desired number of repetitions.

SINGLE ARM ROW

Row kettlebell with one arm, keep other hand free.

1. Stand with feet shoulder-width apart, holding a kettlebell in your right hand.
2. Hinge at your hips, keeping your back straight and knees slightly bent.
3. Row the kettlebell to your right hip, keeping your elbow close to your body.
4. Lower the kettlebell back to the starting position.
5. Repeat for the desired number of repetitions.
6. Switch hands and repeat the movement.

SINGLE ARM SWING

Swing kettlebell with one hand, switch hands mid-air.

1. Stand with feet shoulder-width apart, holding a kettlebell in your right hand.
2. Hinge at your hips, swinging the kettlebell back between your legs.
3. Drive your hips forward to swing the kettlebell up to shoulder height.
4. At the top of the swing, switch the kettlebell to your left hand.
5. Allow the kettlebell to swing back down between your legs.
6. Repeat, alternating hands at the top of each swing.

SINGLE LEG DEADLIFT

Deadlift on one leg holding kettlebell for balance.

1. Stand on your right leg, holding a kettlebell in your left hand.
2. Hinge at your hips, extending your left leg back and lowering the kettlebell towards the ground.
3. Keep your back straight and core engaged.
4. Return to the starting position by driving through your right heel.
5. Repeat for the desired number of repetitions.
6. Switch legs and repeat the movement.

SINGLE LEG ROW

Row kettlebell while standing on one leg.

1. Stand on your right leg, holding a kettlebell in your left hand.
2. Hinge at your hips, extending your left leg back and lowering the kettlebell towards the ground.
3. Row the kettlebell to your left hip, keeping your back straight.
4. Lower the kettlebell back to the starting position.
5. Repeat for the desired number of repetitions.
6. Switch legs and repeat the movement.

SNATCH

1. Stand with feet shoulder-width apart, a kettlebell between your feet.
2. Bend at the hips and knees to grab the kettlebell with one hand.
3. Explosively drive through your heels, pulling the kettlebell upwards.
4. As the kettlebell reaches chest height, flip your wrist and punch upward.
5. Lock your arm overhead, ensuring the kettlebell is stable.
6. Lower the kettlebell back to the starting position and repeat.

Lift kettlebell overhead in one motion, lock arm.

SQUAT

1. Stand with feet shoulder-width apart, holding a kettlebell at chest level or between your legs.
2. Engage your core and squat down, pushing your hips back.
3. Lower your body until your thighs are parallel to the ground.
4. Keep your chest up and back straight throughout the movement.
5. Push through your heels to return to the starting position.
6. Repeat, maintaining proper form.

Squat holding kettlebell at chest or between legs.

SQUAT FLIP

1. Stand with feet shoulder-width apart, holding a kettlebell at chest level.
2. Squat down, keeping the kettlebell stable.
3. As you stand up, flip the kettlebell at chest level, catching it with both hands.
4. Return to the starting position and repeat the movement.
5. Ensure the flip is controlled and smooth.
6. Focus on keeping your core engaged and back straight.

Squat, flip kettlebell at chest level during stand.

STRAIGHT ARM SIT

1. Lie on your back with legs extended, holding a kettlebell with both hands above your chest.
2. Engage your core and sit up, keeping your arms extended straight.
3. Reach a seated position with the kettlebell above your head.
4. Slowly lower back down to the starting position.
5. Maintain straight arms and a stable kettlebell throughout the movement.
6. Repeat, focusing on controlled movements.

Sit-up with arms straight holding kettlebell.

STRETCHING

Use kettlebell for support or resistance during stretches.

1. Use a kettlebell for support or resistance during various stretches.
2. Perform seated stretches with the kettlebell for added resistance.
3. Use the kettlebell to assist in deepening your stretches.
4. Incorporate the kettlebell into dynamic stretches for improved flexibility.
5. Ensure each stretch is held for 20-30 seconds.
6. Repeat each stretch, focusing on maintaining proper form.

SUMO HIGH PULL

Wide-stance pull kettlebell to chin, elbows high.

1. Stand with feet wider than shoulder-width apart, toes pointed outward.
2. Hold a kettlebell with both hands, arms extended downwards.
3. Lower into a sumo squat, keeping your back straight and chest up.
4. Explosively stand up, pulling the kettlebell to your chin.
5. Keep your elbows high and out during the pull.
6. Lower the kettlebell back down and repeat the movement.

Thruster

Squat to overhead press, one fluid motion with kettlebell.

1. Stand with feet shoulder-width apart, holding a kettlebell at chest level.
2. Squat down, keeping your chest up and back straight.
3. As you stand up, press the kettlebell overhead in one fluid motion.
4. Lower the kettlebell back to chest level and repeat.
5. Ensure the transition from squat to press is smooth.
6. Maintain a strong core and stable kettlebell throughout the exercise.

Torso Twist

Stand, twist torso holding kettlebell across body.

1. Stand with feet shoulder-width apart, holding a kettlebell with both hands.
2. Extend your arms in front of you at chest level.
3. Twist your torso to the right, bringing the kettlebell to your side.
4. Return to the center and twist to the left.
5. Keep your hips facing forward and core engaged.
6. Repeat the twisting motion, focusing on controlled movements.

Tricep Dip

Dip using parallel bars, hold kettlebell for added weight.

1. Position yourself between parallel bars, holding a kettlebell with your feet.
2. Lower your body by bending your elbows until your upper arms are parallel to the ground.
3. Keep your elbows close to your body and your core engaged.
4. Push through your palms to extend your elbows and return to the starting position.
5. Repeat, maintaining a controlled movement throughout.
6. Focus on engaging your triceps during the dip.

Tricep Extension

Extend arms overhead, kettlebell in hands.

1. Stand with feet shoulder-width apart, holding a kettlebell with both hands.
2. Extend your arms overhead, keeping your elbows close to your head.
3. Lower the kettlebell behind your head by bending your elbows.
4. Engage your triceps to lift the kettlebell back to the starting position.
5. Keep your core tight and avoid arching your back.
6. Repeat, ensuring controlled movements.

Turkish Get Up

Stand from floor, kettlebell overhead, controlled motion.

1. Lie on your back with your right leg bent and right foot flat on the floor, holding a kettlebell in your right hand.
2. Extend your left arm and leg on the floor.
3. Press the kettlebell straight up, keeping your eyes on it.
4. Roll onto your left forearm, then onto your left hand.
5. Push through your right foot to lift your hips off the ground.
6. Sweep your left leg under your body to a kneeling position.
7. Stand up fully, keeping the kettlebell overhead.
8. Reverse the steps to return to the starting position.
9. Repeat on the other side.

Weighted Lunge

① ②

Lunge holding kettlebell to increase resistance.

1. Stand with feet shoulder-width apart, holding a kettlebell in your right hand.
2. Step forward with your left foot and lower your hips, bending both knees to 90 degrees.
3. Keep your back straight and core engaged.
4. Push through your left heel to return to the starting position.
5. Repeat on the right leg, holding the kettlebell in your left hand.
6. Focus on keeping your weight evenly distributed and maintaining balance.

Windmill

① ②

Reach toward floor, one arm overhead holding kettlebell.

1. Stand with feet shoulder-width apart, holding a kettlebell in your right hand overhead.
2. Turn your left foot out slightly and push your hips to the right.
3. Lower your torso towards the floor, keeping your right arm extended overhead.
4. Reach your left hand towards the ground, keeping your gaze on the kettlebell.
5. Engage your core to return to the starting position.
6. Repeat on the other side, switching the kettlebell to your left hand.

Wood Chop

① ②

Swing kettlebell diagonally across body, squat to lift.

1. Stand with feet shoulder-width apart, holding a kettlebell with both hands.
2. Swing the kettlebell diagonally across your body, starting from your left hip.
3. Squat down slightly as you swing the kettlebell up and across to the right.
4. Engage your core and rotate your torso during the movement.
5. Reverse the motion, bringing the kettlebell back to your left hip.
6. Repeat, focusing on a smooth, controlled motion.
7. Switch sides after completing the desired number of repetitions.

Body-Weight Exercises

Alternate Arm/Leg Plank

Plank, extend opposite arm and leg, hold.

1. Start in a plank position with hands directly under shoulders.
2. Simultaneously lift and extend your right arm and left leg.
3. Hold this position for a few seconds.
4. Return to the plank position.
5. Repeat with the left arm and right leg.

Army Crawl

Crawl flat on stomach, using elbows and knees.

1. Lie flat on your stomach with elbows bent and hands directly in front of you.
2. Push with your toes and pull with your elbows to crawl forward.
3. Keep your body low and hips down.
4. Continue crawling for the desired distance or time.

Back Bridge

Plank, extend opposite arm and leg, hold.

1. Lie on your back with knees bent and feet flat on the floor.
2. Place your hands palms down by your sides.
3. Press through your feet and lift your hips up towards the ceiling.
4. Hold this position, squeezing your glutes and keeping your core tight.
5. Lower your hips back down to the starting position.

Bear Crawl

Crawl forward on all fours, hips down, move quickly.

1. Start on all fours with hands under shoulders and knees under hips.
2. Lift your knees slightly off the ground, keeping your back flat.
3. Move your right hand and left foot forward simultaneously.
4. Follow with your left hand and right foot, maintaining a low position.
5. Continue moving forward in this manner quickly.

Bicycle Crunches

Lie down, alternate elbows to opposite knees cycling legs.

1. Lie on your back with hands behind your head and knees bent.
2. Lift your shoulders off the ground and bring your right elbow towards your left knee while extending the right leg.
3. Switch sides, bringing your left elbow towards your right knee while extending the left leg.
4. Continue alternating sides in a pedaling motion.

Bird Dog

Extend opposite arm and leg, kneeling position.

1. Start on all fours with hands under shoulders and knees under hips.
2. Extend your right arm forward and your left leg backward simultaneously.
3. Hold for a few seconds, keeping your core engaged.
4. Return to the starting position.
5. Repeat with the left arm and right leg.

Bodyweight Row

Pull body up towards a bar or table, lying underneath.

1. Position yourself under a bar or table, gripping it with both hands.
2. Keep your body straight and pull your chest up towards the bar.
3. Hold for a moment at the top of the movement.
4. Lower yourself back down to the starting position.
5. Repeat for the desired number of repetitions.

Burpee

Jump, squat down, kick back into a push-up, return up.

1. Start standing with feet shoulder-width apart.
2. Drop into a squat position and place your hands on the ground.
3. Kick your feet back into a push-up position and lower your body to the ground.
4. Push back up to the push-up position and jump your feet back to your hands.
5. Explosively jump into the air, reaching your arms overhead.
6. Land softly and repeat.

Calf Raise

Raise heels off ground, balance on toes, lower slowly.

1. Stand with feet hip-width apart on a flat surface or step.
2. Lift your heels off the ground, balancing on the balls of your feet.
3. Hold the position for a second.
4. Slowly lower your heels back to the ground.
5. Repeat for the desired number of repetitions.

Calf Raises

Lift heels off ground, balance on toes, lower slowly.

1. Stand with feet hip-width apart on a flat surface or step.
2. Lift your heels off the ground, balancing on the balls of your feet.
3. Hold the position for a second.
4. Slowly lower your heels back to the ground.
5. Repeat for the desired number of repetitions.

Cat/Camel

On hands and knees, arch back up and down.

1. Start on all fours with hands under shoulders and knees under hips.
2. Arch your back up towards the ceiling (Cat position).
3. Hold for a few seconds.
4. Lower your back down and lift your head and tailbone up (Camel position).
5. Alternate between the two positions, moving slowly and smoothly.

Crab Toe Touch

Crawl forward on all fours, hips down, move quickly.

1. Sit on the ground with knees bent, feet flat, and hands behind you.
2. Lift your hips off the ground into a crab position.
3. Reach your right hand to touch your left foot while lifting it.
4. Return to the starting position.
5. Repeat with the left hand and right foot, alternating sides.

Crab Walk

Walk backward on hands and feet, hips elevated.

1. Sit on the ground with knees bent, feet flat, and hands behind you.
2. Lift your hips off the ground into a crab position.
3. Walk backward using your hands and feet, keeping hips elevated.
4. Continue for the desired distance or time.

Crocodile Crawl

Crawl forward lying almost flat, use elbows and toes.

1. Start in a plank position with elbows bent and body low to the ground.
2. Move forward by simultaneously pulling with one arm and pushing with the opposite leg.
3. Keep your body as low and flat as possible.
4. Continue crawling forward for the desired distance or time.

Cross-Body Crunch

Touch opposite knee to elbow, lying down.

1. Lie on your back with knees bent and hands behind your head.
2. Lift your shoulders off the ground and bring your right elbow towards your left knee while extending the right leg.
3. Return to the starting position.
4. Repeat with the left elbow towards the right knee, alternating sides.

Crunch

Lift shoulders off ground, contract abdominals.

1. Lie on your back with knees bent and feet flat on the ground.
2. Place your hands behind your head without pulling on your neck.
3. Lift your shoulders off the ground by contracting your abdominal muscles.
4. Hold for a second at the top.
5. Slowly lower back down to the starting position.

Dolphin Kick

Lie face down, kick legs like a dolphin's tail.

1. Lie face down on a bench with your hips at the edge.
2. Hold onto the bench for support.
3. Lift your legs off the ground, keeping them straight.
4. Kick your legs up and down like a dolphin's tail.
5. Continue for the desired number of repetitions or time.

Donkey Kicks

On hands and knees, kick one leg back and up.

1. Start on all fours with hands under shoulders and knees under hips.
2. Keep your right knee bent and lift your right leg up towards the ceiling.
3. Squeeze your glutes at the top.
4. Lower your leg back down without touching the ground.
5. Repeat on the other leg.

Fire Hydrant

On hands and knees, lift leg to side, keep knee bent.

1. Start on all fours with hands under shoulders and knees under hips.
2. Keep your right knee bent and lift it out to the side.
3. Hold for a moment at the top.
4. Lower your knee back down without touching the ground.
5. Repeat on the other leg.

Flutter Kicks

Lie on back, alternately kick legs in small, rapid motion.

1. Lie on your back with hands under your hips for support.
2. Lift both legs off the ground slightly.
3. Alternately kick your legs up and down in a small, rapid motion.
4. Keep your core engaged and back flat on the ground.
5. Continue for the desired time.

Glute Bridge

Lift hips while lying on back, feet flat on ground.

1. Lie on your back with knees bent and feet flat on the ground.
2. Place your arms by your sides with palms down.
3. Lift your hips towards the ceiling by squeezing your glutes.
4. Hold for a moment at the top.
5. Lower your hips back to the starting position.

Good Morning

Hinge at hips with hands behind head, focus on hamstrings.

1. Stand with feet shoulder-width apart and hands behind your head.
2. Keep your back straight and hinge at the hips, bending forward.
3. Lower your torso until it's parallel to the ground.
4. Focus on feeling the stretch in your hamstrings.
5. Return to the starting position by engaging your glutes and hamstrings.

Hanging Knee Raise

Hang from bar, raise knees towards chest.

1. Hang from a bar with arms extended and feet off the ground.
2. Keep your legs straight and together.
3. Lift your knees towards your chest by engaging your core.
4. Hold for a moment at the top.
5. Lower your legs back to the starting position.

High Knees

Run in place lifting knees high, maintain pace.

1. Stand with feet hip-width apart.
2. Run in place, lifting your knees as high as possible.
3. Pump your arms in coordination with your legs.
4. Maintain a quick pace and keep your core engaged.
5. Continue for the desired time.

Hip Raise

Lift hips while lying on back, feet flat on ground.

1. Lie on your back with knees bent and feet flat on the ground.
2. Place your arms by your sides with palms down.
3. Lift your hips towards the ceiling by squeezing your glutes.
4. Hold for a moment at the top.
5. Lower your hips back to the starting position.
6. Repeat for the desired number of repetitions.

Inchworm

Walk hands forward from standing, hold plank, walk back.

1. Stand with feet hip-width apart.
2. Bend at the waist and place your hands on the ground.
3. Walk your hands forward until you are in a plank position.
4. Hold the plank for a few seconds.
5. Walk your hands back towards your feet and stand up.
6. Repeat for the desired number of repetitions.

Jumping Jacks

Jump to spread legs and clap hands overhead.

1. Stand with feet together and arms at your sides.
2. Jump to spread your legs while raising your arms overhead to clap.
3. Jump back to the starting position with feet together and arms at your sides.
4. Maintain a quick pace and keep your movements controlled.
5. Repeat for the desired number of repetitions or time.

Leg Pull-In

Sit, pull knees into chest, extend legs out.

1. Sit on the ground with legs extended and hands behind you for support.
2. Lean back slightly and lift your legs off the ground.
3. Pull your knees into your chest.
4. Extend your legs back out without touching the ground.
5. Repeat for the desired number of repetitions.

Lunge

Step forward, lower hips to drop knee to ground.

1. Stand with feet hip-width apart.
2. Step forward with your right leg and lower your hips to drop your right knee towards the ground.
3. Ensure your right knee is directly above your ankle.
4. Push through your right heel to return to the starting position.
5. Repeat with the left leg, alternating sides.

Lying Leg Lift

Raise legs vertically, lying flat on back.

1. Lie flat on your back with legs extended and arms by your sides.
2. Keep your legs straight and lift them towards the ceiling until they form a 90-degree angle with your torso.
3. Hold for a moment at the top.
4. Lower your legs back down without touching the ground.
5. Repeat for the desired number of repetitions.

Mountain Climber

Run in place in plank position, drive knees to chest.

1. Start in a plank position with hands under shoulders and body in a straight line.
2. Bring your right knee towards your chest.
3. Quickly switch legs, bringing your left knee towards your chest while extending your right leg back.
4. Continue alternating legs in a running motion.
5. Maintain a quick pace and keep your core engaged.

Pike Push Up

Push-up with hips high, resembles downward dog pose.

1. Start in a downward dog position with hips high and hands shoulder-width apart.
2. Lower your head towards the ground by bending your elbows.
3. Push through your hands to return to the starting position.
4. Keep your body in an inverted V shape throughout the movement.
5. Repeat for the desired number of repetitions.

Plank Rotation

Rotate body in plank, extend arm upward, switch sides.

1. Stand with feet hip-width apart.
2. Step forward with your right leg and lower your hips to drop your right knee towards the ground.
3. Ensure your right knee is directly above your ankle.
4. Push through your right heel to return to the starting position.
5. Repeat with the left leg, alternating sides.

Pull Up

Pull body up on bar, chin above hands.

1. Hang from a pull-up bar with hands shoulder-width apart and palms facing away.
2. Engage your core and pull your body up until your chin is above the bar.
3. Hold for a moment at the top.
4. Lower yourself back down to the starting position with control.
5. Repeat for the desired number of repetitions.

Push Up

Lower body to ground, push up with arms.

1. Start in a plank position with hands slightly wider than shoulder-width apart.
2. Lower your body towards the ground by bending your elbows.
3. Keep your body in a straight line from head to heels.
4. Push through your hands to return to the starting position.
5. Repeat for the desired number of repetitions.

Push-Back

Push body back from push-up position to heels.

1. Start in a plank position with hands under shoulders.
2. Push your hips back towards your heels while keeping your arms extended.
3. Lower your chest towards the ground.
4. Return to the starting plank position.
5. Repeat for the desired number of repetitions.

Push-Up w/ Extension

Perform push-up, extend one arm forward, alternate.

1. Start in a plank position with hands under shoulders.
2. Perform a push-up by lowering your body to the ground.
3. As you push back up, extend your right arm forward.
4. Return your hand to the ground.
5. Repeat with the left arm, alternating sides.

Reverse Crunch

Lift hips off floor, knees towards chest.

1. Lie on your back with knees bent and feet flat on the ground.
2. Place your hands by your sides or under your hips for support.
3. Lift your hips off the ground and bring your knees towards your chest.
4. Hold for a moment at the top.
5. Lower your hips back to the starting position.
6. Repeat for the desired number of repetitions.

Reverse Plank

Sit, lift body with arms, legs straight, face up.

1. Sit on the ground with legs extended and hands behind you, fingers pointing forward.
2. Lift your hips off the ground by pressing through your hands and heels.
3. Keep your body in a straight line from head to heels.
4. Hold for the desired time.
5. Lower your hips back to the ground.

Russian Twist

Twist torso holding weight, seated on ground.

1. Sit on the ground with knees bent and feet flat.
2. Lean back slightly and lift your feet off the ground, balancing on your sit bones.
3. Hold a weight with both hands and twist your torso to the right, bringing the weight beside your hip.
4. Twist to the left, bringing the weight to the other side.
5. Continue alternating sides for the desired number of repetitions.

Scissor Kick

Alternately lift legs in lying position, engages core.

1. Lie flat on your back with hands under your hips for support.
2. Lift your legs slightly off the ground.
3. Alternately lift one leg higher while lowering the other leg, keeping both legs straight.
4. Continue the scissor motion, engaging your core throughout.
5. Repeat for the desired number of repetitions or time.

Side Crunches

Lie on side, perform crunches towards elevated leg.

1. Lie on your side with legs bent and hands behind your head.
2. Lift your upper body towards your hips, crunching towards the elevated leg.
3. Squeeze your obliques at the top of the movement.
4. Lower back down to the starting position.
5. Repeat for the desired number of repetitions, then switch sides.

Side Lunge

Step to side into lunge, keep other leg straight.

1. Stand with feet hip-width apart.
2. Step to the side with your right leg, lowering your hips into a lunge.
3. Keep your left leg straight and your chest up.
4. Push through your right foot to return to the starting position.
5. Repeat on the other side, alternating legs.

Side Plank

Support body on one arm, side facing ground.

1. Lie on your side with your elbow directly under your shoulder.
2. Lift your hips off the ground, forming a straight line from head to feet.
3. Hold this position, keeping your core engaged.
4. For added difficulty, extend your top arm towards the ceiling.
5. Repeat on the other side.

Side-to-Side Pull-Up

Pull up and move sideways along bar, alternate sides.

1. Hang from a pull-up bar with hands shoulder-width apart.
2. Pull your body up towards the bar, moving to the right side.
3. Lower yourself back down and pull up again, moving to the left side.
4. Continue alternating sides.
5. Repeat for the desired number of repetitions.

Side-to-Side Push-Up

Shift side-to-side during push-ups, engages core.

1. Start in a plank position with hands slightly wider than shoulder-width apart.
2. Lower your body towards the ground, shifting your weight to the right.
3. Push back up and shift your weight to the left.
4. Continue alternating sides with each push-up.
5. Repeat for the desired number of repetitions.

Single Leg Dead Lift

Balance on one leg, hinge forward, extend free leg back.

1. Stand on your right leg with a slight bend in the knee.
2. Hinge at the hips, extending your left leg back and lowering your torso towards the ground.
3. Keep your back straight and core engaged.
4. Return to the starting position by squeezing your glutes.
5. Repeat on the other leg, alternating sides.

Single Leg Split Squat

Perform split squat on one leg, elevated rear foot.

1. Stand a few feet in front of a bench or elevated surface.
2. Place your right foot behind you on the bench.
3. Lower your hips into a squat, keeping your left knee over your ankle.
4. Push through your left heel to return to the starting position.
5. Repeat on the other leg, alternating sides.

Single Leg Squat

Stand on one leg, squat, maintain balance.

1. Stand on your right leg, extending your left leg in front.
2. Lower your hips into a squat, keeping your left leg elevated.
3. Maintain balance and keep your chest up.
4. Push through your right heel to return to the starting position.
5. Repeat on the other leg, alternating sides.

Skater Squat

Balance on one leg, squat, touch opposite hand to foot.

1. Balance on your right leg, bending your left knee.
2. Lower into a squat while reaching your left hand towards your right foot.
3. Keep your back straight and chest up.
4. Push through your right heel to return to the starting position.
5. Repeat on the other leg, alternating sides.

Spiderman

Bring knee to elbow during push-up, switch sides.

1. Start in a push-up position with hands under shoulders.
2. Lower your body towards the ground while bringing your right knee to your right elbow.
3. Push back up to the starting position.
4. Repeat with the left knee to the left elbow, alternating sides.
5. Continue for the desired number of repetitions.

Squat

Stand, bend knees to lower body, keep back straight.

1. Stand with feet shoulder-width apart and arms extended in front.
2. Bend your knees and lower your hips into a squat.
3. Keep your back straight and chest up.
4. Push through your heels to return to the starting position.
5. Repeat for the desired number of repetitions.

Star Plank

Extend arms and legs out from body in plank position.

1. Start in a plank position with hands under shoulders and feet together.
2. Extend your right arm and left leg out to the sides.
3. Hold for a moment, keeping your core engaged.
4. Return to the starting position and repeat with the left arm and right leg.
5. Alternate sides for the desired number of repetitions.

Step Up

Step onto a raised platform, alternate legs.

1. Stand in front of a raised platform or bench.
2. Step up with your right foot, bringing your left knee towards your chest.
3. Step back down with your left foot, then your right foot.
4. Repeat with the left foot leading, alternating sides.
5. Continue for the desired number of repetitions.

Stretching

Perform various stretches to improve flexibility and cool down.

1. Perform a variety of stretches, targeting all major muscle groups.
2. Hold each stretch for 15-30 seconds.
3. Focus on slow, controlled movements to increase flexibility.
4. Include stretches for the hamstrings, quadriceps, calves, chest, back, and shoulders.
5. Ensure a thorough cool-down to aid in recovery.

Sumo Squat

Wide stance squat, toes pointed out, lower body.

1. Stand with feet wider than shoulder-width apart and toes pointed out.
2. Lower your hips into a squat, keeping your back straight and chest up.
3. Ensure your knees track over your toes.
4. Push through your heels to return to the starting position.
5. Repeat for the desired number of repetitions.

Superman

Extend arms and legs while face down, hold position.

1. Lie face down on the ground with arms extended forward and legs straight.
2. Lift your arms, chest, and legs off the ground simultaneously.
3. Hold the top position for a few seconds.
4. Lower back down to the starting position.
5. Repeat for the desired number of repetitions.

Swimmer

Lie face down, alternate lifting arms and legs.

1. Lie face down on the ground with arms extended forward and legs straight.
2. Lift your right arm and left leg off the ground simultaneously.
3. Lower them back down and lift your left arm and right leg.
4. Continue alternating sides in a swimming motion.
5. Repeat for the desired number of repetitions or time.

Tricep Dip

Dip body between bars, focus on triceps.

1. Sit on the edge of a bench or chair with hands gripping the edge.
2. Slide your hips off the edge, supporting your weight with your arms.
3. Lower your body by bending your elbows to a 90-degree angle.
4. Push through your palms to return to the starting position.
5. Repeat for the desired number of repetitions.

Tricep Push Up

Push-up with hands under shoulders, elbows tight.

1. Start in a plank position with hands under shoulders and elbows close to your body.
2. Lower your body towards the ground, keeping elbows tight to your sides.
3. Push through your palms to return to the starting position.
4. Keep your body in a straight line throughout the movement.
5. Repeat for the desired number of repetitions.

Tuck Jumps

Jump high, tuck knees to chest mid-air.

1. Stand with feet hip-width apart and knees slightly bent.
2. Jump explosively, bringing your knees towards your chest.
3. Land softly on the balls of your feet with knees slightly bent.
4. Immediately jump again, maintaining quick, controlled movements.
5. Repeat for the desired number of repetitions or time.

V Up

Lie back, lift legs and torso simultaneously, form 'V'.

1. Lie on your back with arms extended overhead and legs straight.
2. Simultaneously lift your legs and torso off the ground, reaching your hands towards your feet.
3. Form a "V" shape with your body at the top of the movement.
4. Lower back down to the starting position with control.
5. Repeat for the desired number of repetitions.

Walking Lunge

Step forward into a lunge, move forward alternating legs.

1. Stand with feet hip-width apart and hands on your hips.
2. Step forward with your right leg, lowering into a lunge.
3. Push through your right heel to stand and bring your left leg forward into the next lunge.
4. Continue alternating legs, moving forward with each step.
5. Repeat for the desired number of repetitions or distance.

Walking Toe Touches

Walk, reach down to touch toes with opposite hand.

1. Stand with feet hip-width apart.
2. Step forward with your right leg, lifting it straight in front of you.
3. Reach your left hand to touch your right toes.
4. Lower your leg and step forward with your left leg, reaching your right hand to your left toes.
5. Continue alternating sides as you walk forward.

Wall Sit

Sit against wall, legs at 90 degrees, hold position.

1. Stand with your back against a wall.
2. Slide down the wall until your thighs are parallel to the ground.
3. Keep your feet shoulder-width apart and knees at a 90-degree angle.
4. Hold this position for the desired amount of time.
5. Maintain tension in your thighs and keep your back flat against the wall.

Wall Squat

Lie face down, alternate lifting arms and legs.

1. Stand with your back against a wall, feet shoulder-width apart.
2. Slide down into a squat position, keeping your back against the wall.
3. Ensure your thighs are parallel to the ground and knees are above your ankles.
4. Hold this position for the desired time.
5. Maintain proper form by keeping your back straight and core engaged.

Wide/Narrow Push Up

Perform push-ups with varying hand widths.

1. Start in a plank position with hands wider than shoulder-width apart.
2. Lower your body to the ground by bending your elbows.
3. Push through your palms to return to the starting position.
4. Move your hands closer together, directly under your shoulders.
5. Perform another push-up in this narrow position.
6. Alternate between wide and narrow push-ups for the desired repetitions.

Windshield Wiper

Swing legs side-to-side lying down, mimic wiper.

1. Lie on your back with arms extended out to the sides for support.
2. Lift your legs off the ground and bring them to a 90-degree angle.
3. Slowly lower your legs to the right side, keeping them together.
4. Bring your legs back to the center.
5. Lower your legs to the left side.
6. Continue alternating sides, mimicking a windshield wiper motion.